NEW DIRECTIONS FOR YOUTH DEVELOPMENT

Theory
Practice
Research

fall | 2004

The Transforming Power of Adult-Youth Relationships

Gil G. Noam
Nina Fiore

issue
editors

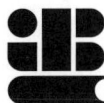

JOSSEY-BASS
A Wiley Imprint
www.josseybass.com

THE TRANSFORMING POWER OF ADULT-YOUTH RELATIONSHIPS
Gil G. Noam, Nina Fiore (eds.)
New Directions for Youth Development, No. 103, Fall 2004
Gil G. Noam, Editor-in-Chief

Microfilm copies of issues and articles are available in 16mm and 35mm, as well as microfiche in 105mm, through University Microfilms Inc., 300 North Zeeb Road, Ann Arbor, Michigan 48106-1346.

NEW DIRECTIONS FOR YOUTH DEVELOPMENT (ISSN 1533-8916, electronic ISSN 1537-5781) is part of The Jossey-Bass Psychology Series and is published quarterly by Wiley Subscription Services, Inc., A Wiley company, at Jossey-Bass, 989 Market Street, San Francisco, California 94103-1741. POSTMASTER: Send address changes to New Directions for Youth Development, Jossey-Bass, 989 Market Street, San Francisco, California 94103-1741.

SUBSCRIPTIONS cost $80.00 for individuals and $170.00 for institutions, agencies, and libraries. Prices subject to change. Refer to the order form at the back of this issue.

EDITORIAL CORRESPONDENCE should be sent to the Editor-in-Chief, Dr. Gil G. Noam, Harvard Graduate School of Education, Larsen Hall 601, Appian Way, Cambridge, MA 02138 or McLean Hospital, 115 Mill Street, Belmont, MA 02478.

Cover photograph © COBIS.

www.josseybass.com

Contents

Editors' Notes

A FUNDAMENTAL SHIFT is occurring in how we view youth and what they need from adults for healthy development. Decades of research and model practices have led up to this moment that is sufficiently significant to be called a paradigm shift. New theories and attitudes, approaches, and practices are beginning to reach many sectors of society—institutions, organizations, and individuals alike. The prevalent mode of dealing with youth has been one of crisis and separation—a model of growth focused on autonomy and on hierarchy between adults and youth. The shift is toward partnership and connection, toward positive youth development and youth voice and responsibility. All of these ways of viewing young people's contributions as extremely important to societal development have to be increasingly embedded in a perspective that young people grow and thrive in relationships and that social institutions, especially families, schools, and youth-serving organizations, have to change to increase their successes. Youth who are connected to adults—parent, teacher, therapist, youth worker, mentor—are far more likely to be resilient, academically successful, and socially adjusted. These relationships serve as protection against adversity, depression, drug use, and school failure. Relationships are even at the core of brain development and neural connectivity.

While a consensus about the significance of relationships between youth and adults is emerging, making the paradigm shift occur, not only in the minds of elites but in the practices of all people, is a more intricate process. This information is absorbed quite differently in different sectors of society. There is very little overlap

NEW DIRECTIONS FOR YOUTH DEVELOPMENT, NO. 103, FALL 2004 © WILEY PERIODICALS, INC.

between the practices of mentors and teachers or between parents and therapists. Some fields, like counseling and psychotherapy, have been undergoing detailed research scrutiny for many years now, while other fields, like youth development, have had relatvely little research input. Youth workers have had a strong relational perspective to work from, whereas therapists have only slowly discovered this perspective through feminist psychology and new psychoanalytical perspectives. Schools, especially at the middle and high school levels, are still in the initial throes of discovering the power and success of a relational perspective, and parents tend to be struggling to embrace such a perspective without falling into a nonproductive, permissive practice. It is time to begin a dialogue across these different sectors and take account of the different languages and needs, the research base, and the theoretical lenses.

As a result of this type of thinking, we began to review the various fields and examine possible areas of overlap. Chapter One highlights our ongoing analysis of these ideas. We opened the discussion to include the other authors in this issue to represent exciting work in multitude fields. All agree that relationships pave the way to positive youth and socioemotional development and academic achievement, but each is handling different issues affecting different relational domains. In Chapter Two, William Pollack addresses the critical role that parent-child relationships and a strong connection to school play in the positive development of youth, especially in avoiding violence, suicidality, and drug abuse. Renée Spencer, in Chapter Three, addresses the connection between the therapist-client relationship and relationships in other contexts, such as mentor-mentee, teacher-student, and practitioner-youth. Katia Fredriksen and Jean Rhodes demonstrate in Chapter Four that the influence and power of the critical parent-child bond can be mimicked and strengthened in the classroom through the role of teachers if the school supports and allows a relational environment. In Chapter Five, Beth Bernstein-Yamashiro presents for the first time her powerful study on teacher-student relationships and their solidifying force during the high school years, and in Chapter Six, Michelle Seligson and Marybeth MacPhee tackle the issue of if, and how, practitioners can be trained to be more relational with their students and thereby reap the most significant student benefits.

This issue of *New Directions for Youth Development* introduces various lenses and shows how much common ground exists and how much work remains. This work is at once exciting and important as we want to create productive environments in which both youth and adults are able to grow together.

We thank our colleagues Sally Wilson, Sara Hoots, Jennifer Levine, Rob McCouch, and the entire PAER and RALLY teams at Harvard and McLean for their contributions to our work and to this issue of *New Directions for Youth Development*. We also thank the Bowne Foundation for support for the work that led to this publication.

Gil G. Noam
Nina Fiore
Editors

GIL G. NOAM, *director of the Program in Afterschool, Education, and Research at Harvard University, is an associate professor of education at the Harvard Graduate School of Education and an associate professor of psychology and director of the Hall-Mercer Laboratory of Developmental Psychology at Harvard Medical School, Boston, and McLean Hospital in Belmont, Massachusetts.*

NINA FIORE *is assistant director of projects and publications at the Program in Afterschool, Education, and Research; a teaching assistant at the Harvard Graduate School of Education; and research coordinator at McLean Hospital/Harvard Medical School.*

Executive Summary

Chapter One: Relationships across multiple settings: An overview

Gil G. Noam, Nina Fiore

Research has shown that students at the most well-attended after-school programs feel bonded to one or more of the adults who work there, that students who feel attached to and respected by their teachers have better academic results, and that patients who feel cared for by their therapist have better therapeutic results. All of these findings show that it is not the method of interaction but the quality of the interaction between patient and therapist, student and teacher, mentee and mentor, youth and youth worker, that is the most critical determinant of success in a myriad of fields.

Chapter Two: Parent-child connections: The essential component for positive youth development and mental health, safe communities, and academic achievement

William S. Pollack

Psychological and developmental models have historically focused on autonomy for youth, and the separation capacity for children, as the hallmark for mental health. This chapter focuses on how those models are not only unhealthy but create premature traumatic disconnections between children or adolescents and their

NEW DIRECTIONS FOR YOUTH DEVELOPMENT, NO. 103, FALL 2004 © WILEY PERIODICALS, INC.

parents. New data illustrate that a continuing parent-youth bond is the foundation for genuine emotional health, academic achievement, and healthy developmental trajectories and also works as an antidote to youth violence.

Chapter Three: Studying relationships in psychotherapy: An untapped resource for youth mentoring

Renée Spencer

Affective bonds and effective collaborations are chronicled in psychotherapy literature as being pivotal to understanding how productive mentoring relationships are formed and sustained, and how such connections foster positive change and development for clients. As we aim to understand more about the intricacies of mentoring relationships in youth development settings, we can turn to psychotherapy to provide keen insight into the essence of strong relationships and their effects on youth.

Chapter Four: The role of teacher relationships in the lives of students

Katia Fredriksen, Jean Rhodes

Warm and supportive teacher relationships have a positive influence on students' academic and psychosocial outcomes. Schools should work to enhance this important bond in order to enable students to reap the many benefits associated with positive student-teacher relationships.

Chapter Five: Learning relationships: Teacher-student connections, learning, and identity in high school

Beth Bernstein-Yamashiro

The study on which this chapter is based reveals that relationships—personal mentoring connections between teachers and students in high school—represent powerful and creative efforts to cross the widening chasm between adults and teenagers in the United States. These relationships are not simply special additions for those who engage in them. Rather, they constitute learning opportunities of their own, unique components of the developmental process, and a potential for community-building at school.

Chapter Six: Emotional intelligence and staff training in after-school environments

Michelle Seligson, Marybeth MacPhee

The goal of applying relational psychology and emotional intelligence to professional development is to foster relationships in which both participants grow. Such relationships offer the recognition, support, and acceptance necessary for developmental change. Adults can find a mix of support and challenge not only in interactions with colleagues and family but also in relationships with children. In fact, caregiving poses a unique developmental challenge: to make meaningful connections with children that are marked by a sense of both responsibility and mutuality.

*The quality and perception of the relationship between
patient and therapist, student and teacher, mentee
and mentor, and youth and youth worker is the most
critical determinant of success in a myriad of fields.*

1

Relationships across multiple settings: An overview

Gil G. Noam, Nina Fiore

WE ARE WITNESSING an underlying shift toward recognizing the
effects of relationships on development for youth and adults alike
in many contexts. Parenting, teaching, mentoring, youth work, out-
of-school programming, and therapy have all had shifts in underlying theory, such as attachment models, resilience studies, and
feminist psychology, toward a focus on the essential role of relationships in growth, learning, and healing.

After-school programs that are well attended, for example, exist
because students feel bonded to one another and to one or more of
the adults who work there.[1] The most academically successful
schools are typically those where students feel attached to and
respected by their teachers.[2] Patients who feel understood and
cared for by their therapist have better therapeutic results.[3] It is not
the specific method of interaction that is the most critical determinant of success in these social fields, whether different styles of
teaching or schools of therapy, but the quality and perception of
the interaction between patient and therapist, student and teacher,
mentee and mentor, youth and youth worker.

NEW DIRECTIONS FOR YOUTH DEVELOPMENT, NO. 103, FALL 2004 © WILEY PERIODICALS, INC.

Such findings are reshaping the way researchers, program developers, and practitioners view and operate within these fields, yet there has still been very little cross-referencing and interdisciplinary work. The desire to spawn cross-pollination stems from the fact that youth typically navigate among these different worlds. In order to assist their development fully, it would help to understand the different relational roles in each sphere of their lives, how they complement one another, and how they can be used to enhance their overall experiences, successes, and life satisfaction. Our own studies[4] suggest that adolescents are especially vulnerable to the fragmentation of interpersonal relationships, social institutions, and interpretative models of understanding reality at a time when the psychosocial task is to create a cohesive and overarching identity.[5] In our words, adolescents benefit from efforts to help them bridge the many worlds they inhabit, institutionally and interpersonally. They have also shown that a sense of belonging plays a critical part in healthy youth-adult development.[6] We believe that this assistance with bridging as well as this sense of belonging is best accomplished through an emphasis on positive, challenging, and supportive relationships.

Resiliency research attests to the overarching significance of adult mentors and role models, especially for young people who face socioeconomic, socioemotional, and educational disadvantage.[7] Relationships formed between students and caring, nonparent adults are invaluable. These relationships allow the students to form attachments to programs, schools, and the community, thus providing a secure base for movement toward a more productive life. Attachment research has shown that positive attachment to more than one person signifies a very primary attachment to the primary caregiver.[8]

However, parent-teacher, parent-therapist, and parent-mentor relationships, among others, are notoriously fraught with misunderstandings. Parents often feel challenged or negated by actions of these other adults[9] and therefore often do not give their children permission, whether conscious or unconscious, to be fully in relationships with teachers, mentors, or counselors. These other adults also frequently ignore parents and thus make an overall investment of the youth in all relationships problematic. We believe that the reason for this is less about personal conflict and more based on institutional understandings of relationships. *Relationship* should not have one definition or be expected to contain the same components within every context.

Another reason to encourage cross-referencing is that the weaknesses of some domains are the strengths of others, and we stand to learn from all of them. Psychology and psychotherapy have the benefit of over fifty years of qualitative and quantitative research into the components of relationships between patients and therapists. These fields have devoted much time and money defining empathy, attunement, and the working alliance that occur during therapy and the resulting effect on the recovery and mental health of patients.[10] Youth development fields such as out-of-school programming and mentoring find their strength in their newcomer status. The limited amount of established, bureaucratic rule allows for a great deal of flexibility and experimentation. Also, given that there is less of a main agenda (in contrast to academic achievement in teaching and recovery in therapy), youth development provides the chance to place relationships at the forefront of its programming and to promote the importance of supportive, encouraging nonparent adults in students' lives. It also provides a testing ground for forging relationships and programming that help students enjoy learning, which helps them build skills.

Attachment theory states that through the earliest interactions between mother (or primary caregiver) and child, the primary attachment model is established.[11] This internal working model of how to relate to another person becomes the foundation for the child's identity and well-being. It also determines the ability the child will have to relate to other people and therefore how secure the child will be about exploring new situations and new topics—in other words, how secure the child will feel about learning and relating—throughout his or her lifetime.[12] Relational psychology furthers this idea by presenting the notion that all learning and development happens as a result of attachments or relationships.

Human beings learn and grow not in isolation but through interactions with one another.[13] Clinical developmental psychology and youth development theory argue that negative internal working models can be modified through the creation of positive internal working models through positive relationships with nonparent adults, such as teachers and mentors.[14] They put forth the idea that teacher-student relationships, for example, may help alter children's negative views of themselves and of others, even if these views have been created through negative family relationships. This means that positive teacher-student relationships could not only boost academic performance but could raise students' overall sense of self and psychological well-being as well.[15] As a result, there is a strong belief in the preventive, restorative, instructive, and developmental power of relationships.

Teachers who form relationships with their students are being presented in research as the most productive. Students respond best to teachers who make them feel "cared about."[16] Awareness of this research and of the successes of some out-of-school programs to motivate learning in students has turned some schools' attention toward what is being done in these programs and how similar methods can be used to improve student participation during the school day. Many schools are realizing that school-age youth in the United States interact with no one else as frequently and consistently as with their teachers on a daily basis and that positive relationships between teachers and students are critical for both student success and the retention of teaching staff. Yet given all its pressures of testing and standards to perform academically, this field has benefited the least from these advances in relational theories.

The problem is societal and institutional as well as individual. There is a willing recognition of the need that younger students have for nurturing, relational environments. However, there is a widely held belief that as students mature, they should develop autonomy to later fully participate in adult society. This is reflected in the design of the school day and its change from a one-teacher classroom in elementary school, to a multiteacher schedule in middle and high school. In the United States, the transition to middle school is a major milestone for the majority of adolescents. Unfortunately, the current school system impersonalizes the school experience in adolescence, right at the time that youth most need support and a sense of belonging. The pressures of pubertal changes and the search for identity are compacted by moving into unfamiliar and often stressful school settings where relationships with teachers are less embedded in the structure than they were in grade school. "Early adolescents' desire for strong relationships with non-parental adults is a poor match with the impersonal halls of large junior high and middle schools where they have less opportunity for positive relationships with their teachers."[17]

Although individual teachers have forged positive relationships with students, most U.S. public, middle, and high schools have not come around to accept a relational point of view. Research has shown that the lack of positive teacher-student relationships is contributing to large student dissatisfaction with schools and teachers and possibly also contributes to teacher burnout.[18]

When many teachers hear the phrase "relationship with students," they imagine their classrooms becoming group therapy forums. This is not at all what we propose here. An attitudinal change toward students is all that is needed for students to pick up on the sense that they are being respected. Given this, most research shows that students will respond in kind. Students have been shown to perform better behaviorally and academically in classes that are taught by teachers who form strong relationships.[19]

Can we train teachers and other practitioners to be relational? In short, we do not think that anyone can be trained to have a different personality, and there are innate qualities that account for easy bonding with students, mentees, and patients. Nevertheless, there are tools that practitioners can use to help them better understand and manage their interactions with youth: "Although many of the emotional, relational and cognitive factors are innate to exceptional practitioners in each field, some of these can be trained and developed further through apprenticeships, work with supervisors, and learning environments that develop these desirable characteristics further in the trainees."[20]

Therapy and counseling have been trying to establish how best to train future therapists to employ not only their cognitive abilities but their emotional and relational ones as well. Multiple studies have shown that it is these emotional and relational factors that contribute to master therapists—those who motivate patients to work on getting well and who have more positive outcomes with their patients than those simply abiding by any one style of therapy and its techniques. With experience and continuous training and supervision, therapists have been found to be better able to bond with patients, intervene effectively, and support their progress. The last decades have seen a strong shift toward making the relationship the central focus of many therapies. The results have been impressive.

We recommend that teachers be trained to develop these relationships with students and, even more important, that schools institutionalize the development and promotion of a relational school climate. Schools need to allow and support teachers in creating supportive classroom environments. They should be aided by mentors and after-school youth workers. In the process, we should not be relying on exceptional personalities alone to carry forward amazing teaching work in adverse contexts. We should be training teachers to handle complicated relationship issues and to make relational growth possible, so they can create important learning relationships with youth. Although we believe that people can and should be trained toward these changes, if institutions do not support and promote such changes, all the training in the world will not help teachers, therapists, mentors, and youth workers. The foundations have been laid in theory, research, and promising practices. Now the institutional changes have to follow.

Notes

1. Miller, B. (2003). *Critical hours: Afterschool programs and educational success.* Quincy, MA: Nellie Mae Education Foundation; Rhodes, J. E., Grossman, J. B., & Resch, N. R. (2000). Agents of change: Pathways through which mentoring relationships influence adolescents' academic adjustment. *Child Development, 71,* 1662–1671.

2. Spencer, R. (2000). *Relationships that empower children for life: A report to the Stone Center directors.* Wellesley, MA: Wellesley College Stone Center. Hamre, B. K., & Pianta, R. C. (2001). Early teacher-child relationships and the trajectory of children's school outcomes through eighth grade. *Child Development, 72,* 625–638; Hughes, J. N., Cavell, T. A., & Jackson, T. (1999). Influence of teacher-student relationship on childhood conduct problems: A prospective study. *Journal of Clinical Child Psychology, 38,* 178–184.

3. Bachelor, A., & Horvath, A. (1999). The therapeutic relationship. In M. Hubble, B. Duncan, & S. Miller (Eds.), *The heart and soul of change: What works in therapy* (pp. 133–178). Washington, DC: American Psychological Association.

4. Noam, G. G. (1999). The psychology of belonging: Reformulating adolescent development. In A. H. Esman, L. T. Flaherty, & H. A. Horowitz (Eds.), *Annals of the American Society of Adolescent Psychiatry* (Adolescent Psychiatry Developmental and Clinical Studies, Volume 24). Hillsdale, NJ: The Analytic Press.

5. Erikson, E. (1968). *Identity and the lifecycle.* New York: Norton.

6. Noam, G. G. (1999, pp. 49–68).

7. Miller. (2003); Pianta, R. C. (1999). *Enhancing relationships between children and teachers.* Washington, DC: American Psychological Association.

8. Bowlby, J. (1969). *Attachment and loss.* New York: Basic Books; Ainsworth, M.D.S. (1989). Attachments beyond infancy. *American Psychologist, 44*(4), 709–716.

9. Rhodes, J. E. (2002). *Stand by me: Risk and rewards of mentoring today's youth.* Cambridge, MA: Harvard University Press. p. 32

10. Luborsky, L. (1994). Therapeutic alliances as predictors of psychotherapy outcomes: Factors explaining the predictive success. In A. O. Horvath & L. S. Greenberg (Eds.), *The working alliance: Theory, research, and practice* (pp. 38–50). New York: Wiley; Horvath, A. O., & Greenberg, L. S. (1989). Development and validation of the working alliance inventory. *Journal of Counseling Psychology, 36,* 223–233; Horvath, A. O., & Symonds, B. D. (1991). Relation between working alliance and outcome in psychotherapy: A meta-analysis. *Journal of Counseling Psychology, 38,* 139–149; Jennings, L., & Skovholt, T. M. (1999). The cognitive, emotional, and relational characteristics of master therapists. *Journal of Counseling Psychology, 46,* 3–11.

11. Bowlby. (1969); Winnicott, D. W. (1965). *The maturational processes and the facilitating environment: Studies in the theory of emotional development.* New York: International Universities Press.

12. Ainsworth. (1989).

13. Rogers, C. R. (1959). A theory of therapy, personality and interpersonal relationships. In S. Koch (Ed.), Psychology: A study of a science (pp. 184–256). New York: McGraw-Hill.

14. Lynch, M., & Cicchetti, D. (1992). Maltreated children's reports of relatedness to their teachers. In R. C. Pianta (Ed.), *Beyond the parents: The role of other adults in children's lives* (pp. 81–107). San Francisco: Jossey-Bass; Pianta, R. C., & Walsh, D. J. (1996). *High-risk children in schools: Constructing sustaining relationships.* New York: Routledge; Noam, G. G., Pucci, K., & Foster, E. (1999). Prevention practice in school settings: The Harvard RALLY

Project as applied developmental approach to intervention with at-risk youth. In D. Cicchetti & S. Toth (Eds.), *Developmental psychopathology: Developmental approaches to prevention and intervention* (pp. 57–109). Rochester, NY: University of Rochester Press; Noam, G. G., & Hermann, C. A. (2002). Where education and mental health meet: Developmental prevention and early intervention in schools. *Development and Psychopathology, 14,* 861–875.

15. Spencer. (2000).

16. Pianta, R. C. (1999).

17. Miller. (2003, p. 10).

18. Poster, M. & Neugebauer, R. (1999). Innovative ideas from the field. In M. L. Culkin (Ed.), *Managing quality in young children's programs: The leader's role.* New York: Teachers College Press, Columbia University.

19. Bernstein, B. L. (1998). *Learning relationships: Teacher-student connections, learning and identity in high school.* Unpublished doctoral dissertation, Harvard University. See Chapter Three, this issue.

20. Jennings & Skovholt. (1999).

GIL G. NOAM, *director of the Program in Afterschool, Education, and Research at Harvard University, is an associate professor of education at the Harvard Graduate School of Education and an associate professor of psychology and director of the Hall-Mercer Laboratory of Developmental Psychology at Harvard Medical School, Boston, and McLean Hospital in Belmont, Massachusetts.*

NINA FIORE *is assistant director of projects and publications at the Program in Afterschool, Education, and Research; a teaching assistant at the Harvard Graduate School of Education; and research coordinator at McLean Hospital/Harvard Medical School.*

Healthy adolescents mature within the context of loving relationships and ongoing connections.

2

Parent-child connections: The essential component for positive youth development and mental health, safe communities, and academic achievement

William S. Pollack

> One of the greatest dignities of humankind is that each successive generation is invested in the welfare of each new generation.
>
> Fred Rogers

IN MAY 1998, at the age of fifteen, Kip Kinkel shot his father and mother to death and the next day opened fire on classmates in Springfield, Oregon, murdering two and injuring twenty-five. He appeared to be a boy from a solid, middle-class family who grew up in a good community. Yet in retrospect, there were aspects of Kinkel's story even those most intimately involved in his life did not appear to know. Whereas school officials and counselors remembered Kip as a likeable teenager not identified as high risk, he soon took the lives of those around him and may well have been contemplating sacrificing his own life as well. Many who were close

NEW DIRECTIONS FOR YOUTH DEVELOPMENT, NO. 103, FALL 2004 © WILEY PERIODICALS, INC.

to him never noticed any warning signs that might indicate potentially self-destructive, violent, or murderous behavior. But there
was a quiet terror and frighteningly ordinary way in which Kip lost
his way and how those who cared about him lost touch with his
eventually lethal pain.

Small, easily unnoticed wounds shaped Kip's interior world: he
was the awkward child in a family that prized athletic prowess, a
boy with a learning disorder in a family of academic achievers, a
boy whose self-esteem was plummeting. And Kip's parents struggled with his overtly growing signs of violence and emotional turmoil. He had become a teenage boy who not only held great inner
pain, but was starting to show outer signs that should have been of
concern to all around him. As he turned into an adolescent, he
became increasingly fascinated with firearms, studied how to make
bombs, and researched small explosives.

Ultimately, as a result of disconnection from all potentially supportive figures around him, he moved to despair. Kip was to write
in his journal prior to the fateful day of the killings, "I am evil and
want to kill and give pain without cost and there is no such thing.
In the end, I hate myself for what I have become."

Am I suggesting that Kinkel is a prototype of all children across
America or his family necessarily typical? Certainly not. However,
the U.S. Secret Service–Department of Education, Safe Schools
Initiative considered forty-one current or recent incidents of such
student attackers.[1] Within these cases of targeted lethal violence at
schools, Kip is more typical than we would like to imagine.

The study found that although planning vicious violence in these
teens' cases varied in its time frame or intricacy, almost all the tragic
events had a lead time from days to months in which some pre-
emptive action could have been taken. Indeed, in a large number
of the cases, the assailant eventually broke his code of silence and
told either a peer or an adult of his intent, but with little or no
interventionary response forthcoming. Most of these tragedies were
preventable early on through the type of community interactions
and connections I describe in this chapter. They were stoppable up
to the last moment if others had only taken proper heed of the seri-
ousness of those youths' communications and had those youths felt

they had a positive connection with someone who could make a difference. But this did not occur. In fact, close to 70 percent of these
so-called killers had been viciously teased or bullied for long periods prior to their violent attacks, and approximately 75 percent had
either threatened suicide or attempted to kill themselves.[2] They
were depressed, and those closest to them did not appear to know
that. Many who used firearms in their attacks took them from their
own families' gun cabinets.

I am not engaging in blame and shame in regard to family structure, for that is the "illness," not the cure. Nor am I trying to over-
sensationalize by choosing an extreme example. I am, however,
attempting to highlight the lack of genuine connection, indeed the
disconnect, between the children and the adults who loved them
and even between the adults in their families and the adults in their
schools who together may have been able to prevent such violence.
Violence, we are learning from our psychological perspective, is
potentially preventable through better support for inter- and
intrafamily relationships.[3] This is not to put the onus on the family or the school, but rather to reempower them as units of safety
and succor and to recognize their myriad opportunities not only to
vouchsafe psychological well-being, but also to prevent the very
troubling aspects of youth violence around us.

New models of connection

The centrality of social-emotional bonds of deep and enduring
meaning, which I refer to as child/youth-adult connections,[4] has
begun to be shown as a central force in the meaningfulness and success of mentorship programs for youth (see Chapter Three, this
volume), antiviolence and antibullying techniques and the creation
of emotional stability in our young,[5] and academic achievement in
the classroom.[6] The core values of adult-youth relationality, however, begin at home, in the cradle of the sustainable and enduring
nidus of parent-child connection. This is an essential bond, both
social-developmental and biologically driven. When it is correctly
and completely provided, it creates the underpinning for our new

models of psychological health for youth beyond the home: as the essential component for healthy child and youth development, academic success, mental stability, and violence-free, safe communities. Such a parent-child connection is at the heart and soul of both the possibility for achievement within programs beyond the home environment and the underpinning of the theories that drive and coordinate new directions for youth in school, after-school programs, sports, mentoring, and rehabilitation. A brief understanding of how we have come to our more modern concept of an evolving but never rupturing parent-child connection as the core of healthy child and youth development deserves both brief description as well as scientific support and qualitative adumbration.

The bedrock of parent-child connection should appear to be a self-evident psychological concept in theory and practice. But only recently has the psychological and psychiatric community been pushed beyond its separation-based models toward these newer and more biosocially reasonable perspectives of ongoing parent-child connection.[7]

For too many years, a confused object-relations model conceptualized separation as the hallmark of mental health.[8] The push for intrapsychic and intrapersonal separation from the mother and other nurturant figures came to be seen as a central normative developmental focus in the healthy growth and development of children and youth. Individuation, or the healthy growth of a sense of self within a context of supportive relationships, became confused with separation, actually the basis for a traumatic abandonment of parental emotional support.[9]

Separation-based atavistic views of children's developmental momentum into adulthood, especially during their adolescent *rites de passage*, have predominated in psychosocial theories of normative development. Along the way, they have taken as hostages not only a vast majority of youth who have been cast into the emotionally disconnected and traumatic Siberia of so-called independence, but particularly the youth groups who have been forced by society into acts of false bravado and violence to prove this death-inducing model of what many psychologists have continued to claim is necessary developmental progress into normative adulthood.

Such belief is not mere speculation. There are both qualitative and interview data drawn from my own extensive interviews with male youths,[10] the growing wave of girl discontent,[11] and a number of larger-scale research samples that point to this central role for adult role modeling and connection in simultaneously sustaining societal health and reducing violence in our midst.

Return to the beginnings

From the perspective of a developmental and clinical psychologist, this brings us to two of the central components that I believe children require from their parenting figures: continuity of attachment, sometimes referred to in the academic literature as *emotional stability*—and what I refer to as stable and loving emotional *connections*—and a dedication to the creation and sustaining of a trusting, loving, nonabusive holding environment that puts these emotional and biological needs first.[12] Winnicott once remarked that "there is no such thing as a baby," meaning that young human primates (whom we psychologists refer to as "children") cannot survive actually or emotionally for any sustained period without what he dubbed as "good enough maternal care." I modify *maternal* to include paternal and partner care. In any case, Winnicott's insight reinforces the significance of healthy psychological attachment as the nexus of what children need from adults and what parents must take on as their primary function.

In moving beyond classical psychoanalytic theories of child development (or perhaps in expanding them), Bowlby and his associates demonstrated through painstaking years of observational study that infants and caretakers require requisite attachments.[13] These opportunities for parent-child connection had sociobiological "prewiring" and occurred in a staged developmental sequence, including growing levels of emotional and cognitive capacity for memory and stabilization. If these "preset" opportunities for caretaker-child interaction did not take place in the proper emotional manner or were significantly disrupted, children would suffer any number of negative behavioral consequences, ranging from delays in emotional development to overt psychopathology, throughout the life cycle.[14] The capacity for caretakers to engage appropriately with these young children required a dedicated set of loving humans, usually parents (but not always so), embedded within a supportive context for both the adults and the offspring: a matrix of positive emotional connections for these caring adults within our society.

Perhaps one of the more unproductive chapters concerning children's development, which I believe we have now begun to put behind us, is the so-called nature versus nurture debate. It is faintly alluded to in Bowlby's pioneering work when he argued for the integration of both biological predispositions and the need for social-interpersonal nurturant interactions. I say "unfortunate," for it has been grounded in a good deal of social scientists' ignorance of modern neurobiology and has also been used by many political zealots to attempt to define these caretaker-child units, which are so essential to children's needs, within a very narrow bandwidth. Then they justified these fallacies with poorly interpreted biological data. My own take on this issue, now widely adopted by the major developmental neurobiologists in the field, is that while children (as well as adults) are "wired for emotional empathic connections," nature requires nurture, and nurture reequilibrates nature. Both are essential in meeting children's needs. Significantly, it does suggest that stable, loving connections are an essential component of parent-child mutuality. These optimal nature-nurture interactions between adults and children provide the support required for optimal child rearing, as well as a positive psychological state required for the adult caretakers themselves.

Modern developmental neurobiology and the potency of parent-child connections

Bruce Perry, a developmental neurobiologist, has declared, "A child's capacity to think, to laugh, to love, to hate, to speak—all of it is a product of *interaction with the environment* [italics added]. Sensory experiences such as touching . . . literally stimulate activity in the brain and the growth of neural structures."[15] Alan Schore, a clinical psychiatrist and biobehavioral scientist, places the central needs of developing children within this context of emotional connection, which I believe the parenting figure must provide and which children require for their physical and mental health: "The idea is that we are born to form attachments, that our brains are physically wired to develop in tandem with another's, through emotional communication, before words are spoken. If things go awry, you're going to see the seeds of psychological problems, of difficulty coping, stress in human relations, substance abuse . . . later on."[16] Caretakers in loving family systems not only affect personality, but do so through direct impact on neural development. Attachments formed within the matrix of a parent-child connection affect young children as people through their developing brain structure: "The self organization of the developing brain occurs within the context of a relationship with another self, another brain. This relational context can be growth-facilitating or growth-inhibiting, and so it imprints into the developing right brain either a resilience against or a vulnerability to forming later psychiatric disorders."[17]

The crisis of childhood and the salience of adult connection

Culled from a basic national survey of close to 100,000 adolescents from grades 7 through 12, Resnick and his colleagues found that what affected adolescent behaviors most was whether their social contexts were mediated by caring adult relationships.[18] According to the study, "parent–family connectedness" dramatically influenced the level of emotional distress adolescents suffer, their level of depression and suicidality, how much they abuse drugs and alcohol, their academic success, general criminal proclivities, and even to some extent how involved in violence they may become. The study also showed other important factors that affect these behaviors, such as whether an adolescent's parents are present during key periods of the day or whether the child's parents have high or low expectations of his or her academic performance. But these factors paled in significance to the connection factor. Such connection, according to the study, involves "closeness to mother and/or father" and a sense of caring emanating from them, as well as "feeling loved and wanted by family members." Indeed, if one parenting figure was positively present within the family, adolescents had two times the protective factors to sustain their health and well-being. If the children felt love or affection from these parents, the protective factor rose to four times.

Resnick's group also found that if adolescents felt connected to an adult who listened to their troubles in the school environment and felt they fit in, there was yet another four times the rise in emotional protectiveness. They found that youth will thrive at school if there is a pervasive sense that they are welcome, that they are liked, and that who they really are—and how they really enjoy learning—is embraced in a genuine way by their teachers. They demonstrated that the largest factor protecting young people from emotional distress, drug abuse and violence—in addition to the closeness they were able to achieve within their families—was "perceived school connectedness."

The more students feel connected, understood, and treated fairly at school, the less likely they are to become suicidal, abuse drugs and alcohol, become addicted to nicotine, or engage in impulsive sexual activities. Youth do best when they feel cared for and understood by their teachers and when they sense that teachers have high hopes for them academically. By designing an inviting (that is, emotionally connected) educational experience for students, schools can help them boost not only their academic performance and self-esteem but also their hopefulness about the opportunities ahead of them. They will not suffer the fate of Kip Kinkel, his classmates, and other adolescents caught up in school violence.[19]

The potency of loving adult-child relationships is much stronger than even the best (and potentially useful) antiviolence program, certainly greater than any simple-minded, required, zero-tolerance curriculum, and more productive and less traumatic than any magnetometer or gun-sniffing dog.

Ongoing family connection: Avoiding disconnection

What I and others have found in research with children as they grow to the teenage years is that what they need most to survive negative peer pressures and the other tribulations of adolescence is knowing that they have meaningful connections with their parents and other significant adults. Although we are often taught that adolescents need or want to separate from their families, this is a dangerous, unsubstantiated myth.[20] Certainly adolescents are struggling with issues of identity and growth and will push at us, even push away from us, at times. Certainly they wish to spend some time away from home and develop an individual, individuated sense of self. But these youngsters rarely wish to cut their ties, be on their own, or separate. In fact, most children desperately need their parents and the extended family—coaches, teachers, clergy—to be there for them, stand firm yet show flexibility, and form a living wall of love that they can lean on—and bounce off—regularly. It is not separation but rather individuation. It is becoming a more mature self in the context of loving relationships and ongoing connections—stretching the psychological umbilical cord rather than severing it—that healthy adolescence is all about.

My own research shows that youth know this only too well. Fifteen-year-old Seth (not his real name), in describing how he copes with the "separation" pain many adolescents experience, replied buoyantly, "I think . . . [it's] just the *closeness* of my family. The way my parents have brought me up to want to be part of the family. I love going home and spending time with my mom or my dad. Sometimes I'd rather be with my family."

Adolescents who know that they have a loving adult and can tap into the strength derived from that positive relationship—the potency of connection—have what they need to make it through adolescence. Again and again in my research, teens refer to the importance of family. I firmly believe that it is the potency of parent-youth connection that guards adolescents from falling prey to violence or emotional harm and gives them the most reassurance in the adolescent world of "cool."

Other psychologists as well have corroborated the central role of family connections during adolescence. Feldman and Wentzel found that the perception youths have of their parents' marital satisfaction directly affected their social adjustment during adolescence.[21] Blake Bowden of the Cincinnati Children's Hospital found that children and adolescents who ate dinner with their family five times a week were least likely to use drugs or be depressed and most likely to excel at school and have a healthy social life.[22] Perhaps the most striking data-based support for this thesis comes from the large-scale University of Minnesota National Longitudinal Study on Adolescent Health, the work of Resnick et al. described earlier. Most recently, in fact, Resnick stated that "the sense of connectedness to adults is salient as a protective factor against any array of health jeopardizing behaviors . . . and has protective effects for both boys and girls across ethnic, racial and social class groups."[23] Such connection, according to the study, involves "closeness to mother and/or father" and a sense of caring emanating from them, as well as "feeling loved and wanted by family members."

The adult's protective value does not come from a sense of being a moral policeman or warden, as some would have us believe, or from a laissez-faire attitude. Rather, it is the potency of adult connection that guards children from emotional harm and gives them succor from a world that is rough, a niche where a youth may express his or her most vulnerable and warm feelings in the open, without fear of ridicule. In return for their protection from harm, we adults are protected from being harmed by violence as a desperate adolescent's last-ditch efforts at connection or despairing protest of disconnection.

Connecting with our youth: Creating genuine bonds of safety and family havens

Psychological data and clinical expertise can provide some useful and timely advice on family policy recommendations:

• *Create and sustain child-oriented parent and caregiver connections.* Create an emotional holding environment early, and do not relinquish it. That is not to say we should smother children, but there is no such thing as loving them *too much*. This creates shame-free zones for talk and emotional safety nets of connection. We need human detectors and protectors, not gun detectors, to provide safety for our youth.

- *Listen.* That means not to lecture but, in the case of more reticent girls and a vast majority of preteen and adolescent boys, to enlarge a wider panoply of skills to include "action talk with listening."[24]
- *Understand behavior as a form of reaching out.* Even the most seemingly negativistic interaction is a moment to capture and transform parent-child activity and ultimately talk. Do not castigate yourself for not being perfect at parenting (be a "good-enough parent"), but never give up either. Blame-free environments at home are good for parent and child. Worry less about limits, and focus on shared human frailty and joy with reality limitations that children and adults both need to face.
- *Do not go it alone.* That is exactly where young people are getting stuck. Whether a traditional mother-father pair, a single parent, or one of the myriad of new family constellations, we need to reach out to like-minded neighbors, clergy, other parents, and schools for the support of connection. Mentors from outside the immediate family network are important for children.

Chaim Ginnott, the great parent educator, used to advise parents of teens that at times of turmoil, "Don't just do something, stand there." Being there is half of the story; showing love is the other half. Youth who have a connection to a caring adult, share meals with them, and feel loved and understood, have higher self-esteem and higher success rates in life, and they are more psychologically resilient. Do not feel as if the weight of the world is all on adult shoulders, but do recognize that the potency of parenting or caregiving has ten times the power of biology or peer culture— not only in making our children's world safer but ultimately in making their lives and ours more joyful and meaningful.

We must work to reframe the small society of our homes and the broader organizational surround into cultures of connection in which adults are willing to relate and listen. Then young people will feel safe to talk not just about impending danger to and from themselves or their peers—building a genuine psychological health nexus—but also about all those deep yearnings for adult guidance. As one boy expressing a ray of hope in his then dark and saddened world told me, "A mother's love transcends all things, and now my dad also talks to me in a way I can talk to him." No list of warning signs, profiles, or judicial interventions can ensure that level of genuine security for both generations and for our society as a whole.

In the first century B.C.E., the great Hebrew scholar Hillel tackled many of the questions we still face at the dawn of the twenty-first century. He asked what the nature and the limits are of our responsibilities as adults to our children and questioned the existential pressures to act. In the end, he argued for a compromise between recognition of individual need and emotional connection or a simultaneous balance between individuation (*not* separation), on the one hand, and what he saw as a spiritual (and what I have argued as a socioneurobiological) reality to remain emotionally bonded, on the other. He not only presaged a good deal of modern psychological debate but framed a question that goes to the heart of this topic: new models for healthy adolescent and child development within connection to parent and other adult caregivers that even in the most fragile social environments will sustain healthy attachment and growth. Translated from the Hebrew, Hillel opined:

If I am not for myself, who will be for me?
But if I am for myself alone, then what am I?
If not now, then when?

Indeed, in creating and maintaining the adult-child connection as the bulwark for a range of new interventional models for healthy youth development and in struggling for the hearts and souls of our youth, we too must ask ourselves, "If not now, then when?"

Notes

1. Fein, R., Vossekuil, B., Pollack, W., Borum, R., Modzeleski, W., & Reddy, M. (2002). *Threat assessment in schools: A guide to managing threatening situations and to creating safe school climates.* Washington, DC: U.S. Department of Education & U.S. Secret Service.

2. Fein et al. (2002).

3. Fein et al. (2002).

4. Although for the majority of the chapter I will refer for the purposes of clarity and space to the parent-child connection, the word *parent* as used in this context is meant to encompass a wide-ranging view of primary home-based caregivers and nurturers who vary dramatically from the Ozzie and Harriet world of biological parent. This compressed term is also meant to recognize simultaneously both the significance of two-parent arrangements of two genders and the scientifically supported significance of both one-parent households with a primary caregiver of either gender or two-parent homes with caregivers of the same gender, as well as so-called blended families. In the same light, the word *child* will often stand for both younger children and older ones more correctly referred to as youth.

At times the broader context of caregiver versus parent or youth or adolescent versus child will find its direct place in the chapter to highlight these points, but those moments should not be read as the only times that this broader perspective is brought to bear. It is at the heart of my larger argument.

5. See Pollack, W. S. (1998). *Real boys: Rescuing our sons from the myths of boyhood.* New York: Random House.

6. Cohen, J. (Ed.). (2001). *Caring classrooms/intelligent schools.* New York: Teachers College Press

7. Pollack, W. S. (1995a). No man is an island: Toward a new psychoanalytic psychology of men. In R. Levant & W. Pollack (Eds.), *A new psychology of men* (pp. 33–67). New York: Basic Books; Pollack, W. S. (1995b). Deconstructing disidentification: Rethinking psychoanalytic concepts of male development. *Psychoanalysis and Psychotherapy, 12*(1), 30–45.

8. M. S. Mahler, F. Pine, & A. Bergman. (1975). *The psychological birth of the human infant.* New York: Basic Books.

9. Pollack. (1995a, 1995b, 1998).

10. Pollack. (1998); Pollack, W. S. (1999). The sacrifice of Isaac: A new psychology of boys and men. *SPSMM Bulletin, 4*, 7–14; Pollack, W. S. (2000). *Real boys' voices.* New York: Random House.

11. Brown, L. M. (2003). *Girlfighting.* New York: NYU Press; Brown, L. M. (1999). *Raising their voices.* Cambridge, MA: Harvard University Press; Prothrow-Stith, D., & Spivak, H. R. (2003). *Murder is no accident.* New York: Wiley.

12. Winnicott, D. W. (1974). *The maturational processes and the facilitating environment.* New York: IUP Press.

13. Bowlby, J. (1969, 1973, 1980). *Attachment and loss* (Vols. 1–3). New York: Basic Books.

14. Robertson, J., & Robertson, J. (1971). Young children in brief separation. *Psychoanalytic Study of the Child, 26*, 264–315.

15. See Pollack. (1998, p. 57).

16. Schore, A. N. (2003). *Affect dysregulation and disorders of the self.* New York: Norton Press, p. xv; Commission on Children at Risk. (2003). *Hardwired to connect.* New York: Institute for American Values, p. xv.

17. Schore. (2003).

18. Resnick, M. D., Bearman, P. S., Blum, R. W., Bauman, K. E., Harris, K. M., Jones, J., Tabor, J., Beuhring, T., Sieving, R. E., Shew, M., Ireland, M.,

Bearinger, L. H., & Udry, J. R. (1997). Protecting adolescents from harm. *Journal of the American Medical Association, 278*(10), 823–832.

19. Pollack. (2000).

20. Pollack, W. S. (2001). *Real boys workbook.* New York: Random House

21. Feldman, S. S., & Wentzel, K. R. (1995). Relations of marital satisfaction to peer outcomes in adolescent boys: A longitudinal study. *Journal of Early Adolescence, 5,* 220—237.

22. Elias, M. (1997. Aug. 15). Family dinners nourish ties with teenagers. *Wall Street Journal.*

23. Commission on Children at Risk. (2003).

24. Pollack. (1998, 1999, 2000).

WILLIAM S. POLLACK *is the director of the Centers for Men and Young Men at McLean Hospital in Belmont, Massachusetts, and assistant clinical professor in the Department of Psychiatry at Harvard Medical School. He is a fellow of the American Psychological Association.*

The core elements of effective psychotherapy may be key ingredients of effective mentoring relationships as well.

3

Studying relationships in psychotherapy: An untapped resource for youth mentoring

Renée Spencer

THE PSYCHOTHERAPY LITERATURE has much to offer as we strive to develop deeper and more nuanced understandings of the relationships youth form with mentors and other nonparental adults in community- and school-based settings. At the center of both psychotherapy and relationship-based interventions such as mentoring is a human connection, the explicit goal of which is to foster positive changes in one of the partners. Attention has long been paid to the nature of this connection in the psychotherapy literature—what it is and should be composed of, how it is best formed and facilitated, and what part it plays in the change process. Although the relationships that youth form with mentors are certainly of a different nature from a psychotherapy relationship, there are some parallels and perhaps even core elements that these different types of important connections share.

To underscore the importance of relationship building in mentoring can sound trite. Few would argue with the assertion that the relationships forged between youth and their mentors shape the nature of the benefits youth derive from these programs. Yet building strong relationships is neither straightforward nor easy, and the

NEW DIRECTIONS FOR YOUTH DEVELOPMENT, NO. 103, FALL 2004 © WILEY PERIODICALS, INC.

field of youth mentoring is only beginning to move beyond stressing that close relationships make a difference to devoting more serious efforts toward delineating how such relationships form and the specific processes through which they promote positive outcomes for youth. Such connections are critical for many youth as changes in our communities, family structure, and work demands are converging to decrease youth's access to ongoing, caring, and close relationships with adults.[1] Mentoring and other programs that link youth with caring and competent adults are sorely needed to fill this growing gap, as adults in these programs often have opportunities to engage with youth in ways that teachers and many overburdened parents are unable. Yet it is also imperative that we move to ensure that the relationships formed through mentoring and other relationship-based programs are high-quality relationships that do indeed help youth in need.

The psychotherapy literature remains a largely untapped resource for more detailed, complex, and sophisticated approaches to understanding how productive relationships are formed and sustained and how such connections foster positive change and development. In this chapter, I review research on the core elements of psychotherapy relationships that work regardless of the theoretical framework being employed. This literature, dense and diffuse though it is, nonetheless clearly highlights two important dimensions of strong relationships that foster change and growth: an affective bond and an effective collaboration.

Common factors in psychotherapy

The psychotherapy field has spawned an estimated more than two hundred theoretical frameworks and an even larger number of accompanying sets of specific techniques.[2] Some of the major approaches that have large followings are cognitive-behavioral, interpersonal, and psychodynamic theories. However, the search for evidence promoting the efficacy of one type of psychotherapeutic treatment over another (say, cognitive-behavioral versus interpersonal) has yielded few consistent differences among modalities.[3] Rather, differences tend to appear within a modality, with some therapists getting consistently better results with their clients than do other therapists using the same approach.[4] Such findings have fueled the search for common factors or core elements of effective therapy that cut across the specific approaches being employed. The common factors that have received the greatest attention[5] are those originally delineated by Rogers[6] in his client-centered approach: empathic understanding, warmth and positive regard, and congruence or authenticity. It is important to note, and potentially instructive for the study of youth-adult relationships, that it is the clients' perception of these aspects of the relationship, rather than observer or therapist measurements, that are more consistently predictive of client outcomes.[7]

Empathy, long a focus of study in the psychotherapy literature, can be thought of most simply as understanding another person's frame of reference and affective experience, or as it is often described more colloquially, stepping into another's shoes.[8] Therapists who are able to do this effectively and without getting overwhelmed themselves retain what Rogers called an "as-if" quality when striving to enter into another's experience that keeps them from getting immersed in their own emotions.[9] Higher levels of perceived therapist empathy have been found to be correlated with a greater likelihood of staying in treatment. It is also considered to be linked with better outcomes in therapy through facilitating feelings of safety, making it more likely the client will self-disclose, promoting meaning making, and activating the client's own self-healing capacities.[10]

A warm acceptance of, or positive regard for, the client on the part of the therapist is thought to be vital to the change process because it communicates to clients that they are of worth and that their thoughts, feelings, opinions, and ideas matter.[11] Furthermore, a general sense of positive regard for the client helps the therapist to consider resistance, apathy, anger, or other manifestations of

challenges and difficulties faced by the client within the larger context of the individual's personhood and desires to learn and connect
with others, helping the therapist to stay connected with the client
during difficult moments in the psychotherapy process. Rogers
believed that people who experience this type of caring will develop
a more caring attitude toward themselves. Reviews of studies linking positive regard to treatment outcomes have found a modest but
consistent association between the two. It has also been suggested
that the presence of positive regard increases the likelihood that
clients will stay in treatment.[12]

Rogers asserted that the therapist's genuine presence in the relationship facilitates change and growth on the part of the client.[13] This
matching, or congruence, of the therapist has two parts: (1) the therapist has the capacity to experience himself or herself with clients in
the therapy hour and (2) is able to communicate these experiences to
clients in an appropriate way. Put another way, the client must not be
left with the sense that the therapist is putting up a facade or playing
a role. This condition is essential to the change process, in Rogers's
view, because in its absence, clients will be cautious and unlikely to
drop their defenses so that learning and growth can occur. Furthermore, the therapist's own genuineness serves as a model and facilitates clients' becoming more open to their own feelings and able to
express these without fear. Findings from studies examining the link
between therapist congruence and client outcomes have been mixed.
However, the methodological challenges posed by this type of
research have led some reviewers of these studies to conclude that a
consistent pattern linking congruence to positive therapy outcomes
suggests that it does play a role in the change process, most likely
working in concert with empathy and positive regard.[14]

Together, empathy, positive regard, and congruence comprise
what has been called the supportive relationship in psychotherapy,
or the positive emotional bond, which serves as the foundation for
the treatment. These ingredients are thought to contribute to the
client's feeling listened to and understood and experiencing the therapist as trustworthy and helpful, without which the therapy stands
little chance of continuing or being effective. Another important

aspect of the therapy relationship is the collaborative, or working, relationship.[15] Therapists who engage their clients in a collaborative, rather than a directive or passive, relationship tend to get better results with their clients.[16] Although this ultimately requires the participation of both client and therapist, some therapists do seem to be better than others at engaging clients in this way.[17]

Recently, researchers have tended to conceptualize both the supportive and collaborative components of the psychotherapy relationship as being part of the therapeutic alliance, embedding the Rogerian ideas into what has been termed a "two-person" field, or one that takes into account the contributions of both therapist and client. Defined in many ways, it is generally thought to comprise (1) the bond between therapist and client, (2) agreement on goals of treatment, and (3) mutual engagement in tasks that facilitate movement toward these goals.[18] The therapist's ability to effectively deal with ruptures in the relationship has also been considered a key aspect of the alliance.[19] The common factors of empathy, congruence, and positive regard are thought to contribute to the formation of the bond between therapist and client. Agreement on goals and collaborative engagement in tasks facilitates the client's acceptance of and adherence to the treatment plan. These two aspects of the working alliance are thought to be interdependent, in that each builds on and facilitates the growth of the other.[20] The quality of the therapeutic alliance, particularly its formation early in the therapy process, has been found to be a powerful and consistent predictor of more effective treatment.[21]

Most of this research on psychotherapy relationship processes and treatment outcomes has been conducted on therapy with adults; however, the little research that has been conducted with youth has yielded similar results. The rise in behavioral treatments for youth, along with the move toward comparisons of specific treatment approaches in psychotherapy outcome research more generally, contributed to a shift in focus away from the therapeutic relationship.[22] More recently, there has been a resurgent interest in the contribution that interpersonal processes make to effective treatment with youth. A recent meta-analysis of twenty-three studies found that the therapeutic relationship is modestly but consistently related to treatment outcomes among youth across diverse types of treatment.[23]

More than thirty years of research and literally hundreds of studies now point to the central importance of the therapy relationship for effective treatment across a wide range of problems. One researcher reviewing this extensive literature attributes most of the systemic variance in psychotherapy outcomes to the alliance that forms between therapist and client.[24] Others are a bit more modest in their assessment, estimating that about 30 percent of the variance in outcomes is attributable to the strength of the bond and working relationship formed and also estimating that specific techniques employed (for example, the use of cognitive restructuring by a cognitive-behavioral therapist) are thought to account for about 15 percent.[25] Both the relationship and the specific approach employed play a role in the therapeutic process; however, the relationship is central to all forms of therapy. Attending to the formation and maintenance of a strong and positive working relationship is clearly a cornerstone of effective psychotherapy.

Implications for youth mentoring

Mentoring, like psychotherapy, is a relationship-based intervention. The intention behind mentoring is to match youth in need with a competent, caring adult in the hopes that a strong and lasting connection will be forged that will facilitate the youth's positive psychological growth and adjustment. Simply being matched with a mentor does not yield these hoped-for benefits; the small but growing empirical base in the youth mentoring field is beginning to call attention to the importance of higher-quality mentoring relationships.[26] Frequent contact over time appears to be important, providing insight into the frame of effective mentoring relationships.[27] In addition, a strong, positive affective bond is emerging as a key ingredient: a young person is more likely to derive positive benefits from mentoring when the relationship is experienced as close and the mentor becomes a significant adult in his or her life.[28] However, the factors that contribute to the development of these strong ties have only begun to be considered.

Although mentoring is not psychotherapy, it is a helping relationship, and it stands to reason that the core elements of effective psychotherapy may be key ingredients of effective mentoring relationships as well. The psychotherapy process research would suggest that mentors should strive to nurture a strong, positive affective bond, particularly in the early stages of the relationship. Adults who are skilled at being empathic with youth, appropriately genuine or authentic in their exchanges, and feel and convey an overall sense of positive regard for the youth are likely to be better able to weather the challenges that may arise as the relationship is taking shape and may be more effective at ultimately building strong connections with youth. Furthermore, this research suggests that mentors should strive to build collaborative working relationships with youth, neither becoming too directive nor allowing youth to become too passive in their exchanges.

Research on youth development, after-school contexts, and mentoring are all beginning to point to the importance of these aspects of growth-promoting adult-youth relationships. Both quantitative and qualitative studies of mentoring relationships have indicated that authenticity, engagement, and empathy are qualities present in effective mentoring relationships.[29] Research on adult-youth relationships in family and after-school settings has suggested that the most effective adults are those who provide a balance of appropriate structure, challenge, and support.[30] Collaborative processes are receiving greater attention in research on cognitive development as well. Building on Vygotsky's ideas, Rogoff has proposed that learning takes place through collaborative participation in shared activities, or what she calls guided participation.[31] Particularly potent seem to be those experiences in which the young person and the more skilled partner focus their joint attention on a task of interest to the youth.[32]

However, in mentoring relationships, as in psychotherapy, the onus lies squarely on the adult to reach out to and engage with the youth in ways intended to meet their needs and foster their development. Not all youth enter mentoring relationships with the same needs. Youth who have enjoyed good relationships with their parents and other supportive adults, for example, may be drawn to adult mentors largely as role models or as guides. In such cases, the relationship may focus more on the acquisition of skills and the advancement of critical thinking than on emotional issues.[33] In these cases, mentors who entered the relationship hoping to serve as a close confidant to a young person may find their mentee more receptive to being exposed to opportunities for learning and new experiences. Other youth who have experienced unsatisfactory or difficult parental ties may develop more intense bonds with available adults to satisfy their social and emotional needs.[34] Some of these youth may even need to form such a bond before they are able or willing to accept other forms of guidance and support from an adult.[35] The psychotherapy literature, particularly more relationally oriented approaches that focus on navigating relational exchanges in ways that facilitate the development of the relationship and foster positive change in the client, could be mined for guidance about how best to approach exchanges with youth, particularly those with histories of troubled relationships.[36]

In addition, differences in backgrounds between adult volunteers and youth may play a role in the development of strong ties in mentoring relationships. Many youth of color in mentoring programs are matched with white mentors, as these youth would remain on long waiting lists if matches were made solely on the basis of race.[37] Thus far, the research examining whether there are differences in the benefits to youth of same- versus cross-race matches has yielded mixed results, with some finding no differences and others finding that cross-race relationships were more likely to end prematurely.[38] In recent years, a key component of psychotherapy training and supervision has been the development of knowledge and skills needed to work effectively with diverse clients, particularly important for professionals who work with clients with racial, ethnic, cultural, and class backgrounds different from their own.[39] This already extensive literature could be examined and tapped for creating more effective training programs for volunteer mentors and for program staff who monitor and assist developing matches.

It should also be stressed that there are limits to the parallels between mentoring and psychotherapy. A mentor is not a psychotherapist, and one of the dangers of drawing on the psychotherapy literature as a knowledge base for youth mentoring may be to overestimate what adults can and should try to accomplish through a mentoring relationship with a young person. Such practices could inadvertently run the risk of harming, rather than helping, already vulnerable youth. Recognizing the limits of the mentoring role and seeking outside guidance and counsel when doubts and uncertainties arise could also prove critical to effective mentoring.

Given that mentoring relationships tend to be more focused on promoting overall development than more remedial change, other factors specific to these types of relationships are also important. For example, mentoring relationships provide opportunities for youth to engage in recreational and more socially focused interactions with adults. Such activities may provide youth a welcome respite from difficult circumstances with which they are faced while also fostering positive bonds and providing enriching learning experiences. The research on social support has begun to highlight engaging in mutually pleasurable social activities as a distinct aspect of supportive relationships, labeling it companionship, and distinguishing it from other forms of social support that are sought out during times of distress.[40] Companionship is motivated by the desire to share in "purely enjoyable interaction, such as the pleasure in sharing leisure activities, trading life stories and humorous anecdotes, and engaging in playful spontaneous activities," and is believed to be a contributor to overall well-being.[41] In qualitative studies of relationships between youth and adults, youth cite being able to have fun and being interested in engaging with them in some of their favorite activities as qualities that distinguish adults with whom they more easily connect.[42] Such shared experiences of companionship may distinguish more effective mentoring relationships.

We would be wise to stand on the broad shoulders of the psychotherapy research literature and begin to augment our developing understanding of the importance of close and enduring mentoring relationships by devoting serious attention to delineating the factors that facilitate the formation of such ties between youth and adults. Such knowledge would provide guidance for more effective training of mentors and help identify critical supports that need to be in place to nurture developing mentoring relationships. The common factors of effective psychotherapy relationships—empathy, positive regard, and congruence—accompanied by a collaborative working relationship are strong candidates for our consideration. In this time of unprecedented mentoring program expansion, the tendency to focus on rapidly matching as many youth as possible with available mentors should be tempered by greater attention to ensuring that the matches that are made are of high quality. The psychotherapy literature provides some solid jumping-off points for consideration of what processes may help to promote the formation of closer and more effective mentoring relationships.

Notes

1. Scales, P. C. (2003). *Other people's kids: Social expectations and American adults' involvement with children and adolescents.* Norwell, MA: Kluwer.

2. Hubble, M. A., Duncan, B. L., & Miller, S. D. (Eds.). (1999). *The heart and soul of change: What works in therapy.* Washington, DC: American Psychological Association.

3. Ahn, H., & Wampold, B. E. (2001). Where oh where are the specific ingredients? A meta-analysis of component studies in counseling and psychotherapy. *Journal of Counseling Psychology, 48*(3), 251–257.

4. Ogles, B. M., Anderson, T., & Lunnen, K. M. (1999). The contribution of models and techniques to therapeutic efficacy: Contradictions between professional trends and clinical research. In M. A. Hubbles, B. L. Duncan, & S. D. Miller (Eds.), *The heart and soul of change: What works in therapy* (pp. 201–225). Washington, DC: American Psychological Association.

5. Lambert, M. J., & Barley, D. E. (2002). Research summary on the therapeutic relationship and psychotherapy outcome. In J. C. Norcross (Ed.), *Psychotherapy relationships that work: Therapist contributions and responsiveness to patients* (pp. 17–32). New York: Oxford University Press.

6. Rogers, C. R. (1959). A theory of therapy, personality and interpersonal relationships. In S. Koch (Ed.), *Psychology: A study of a science* (pp. 184–256). New York: McGraw-Hill.

7. Horvath, A. O., & Symonds, B. D. (1991). Relation between working alliance and outcome in psychotherapy: A meta-analysis. *Journal of Counseling Psychology, 38*(2), 139–149; Wampold, B. (2001). *The great psychotherapy debate: Models, methods, and findings.* Mahwah, NJ: Erlbaum. Lambert & Barley. (2002).

8. Bohart, A. C., Elliott, R., Greenberg, L., & Watson, J. C. (2002). Empathy. In J. C. Norcross (Ed.), *Psychotherapy relationships that work: Therapist contributions and responsiveness to patients* (pp. 89–108). New York: Oxford University Press.

9. Rogers. (1959).

10. Bohart et al. (2002).

11. Rogers, C. R. (1980). *A way of being.* Boston: Houghton Mifflin.

12. Farber, B. A., & Lane, J. S. (2002). Positive regard. In J. C. Norcross (Ed.), *Psychotherapy relationships that work: Therapist contributions and responsiveness to patients* (pp. 175–194). New York: Oxford University Press.

13. Rogers. (1980).

14. Klein, M. H., Kolden, G. G., Michels, J. L., & Chisholm-Stockard, S. (2002). Congruence. In J. C. Norcross (Ed.), *Psychotherapy relationships that work* (pp. 195–215). New York: Oxford University Press.

15. Walborn, F. S. (1996). *Process variables: Four common elements of counseling and psychotherapy.* Pacific Grove, CA: Brooks/Cole.

16. Orlinsky, D. E., & Howard, K. I. (1986). Process and outcome in psychotherapy. In S. L. Garfield & A. E. Bergin (Eds.), *Handbook of psychotherapy and behavior.* New York: Wiley.

17. Walborn. (1996).

18. Horvath, A. O., & Luborsky, L. (1993). The role of therapeutic alliance in psychotherapy. *Journal of Consulting and Clinical Psychology, 61*(4), 561–573.

19. Lambert & Barley. (2002).

20. Horvath & Luborsky. (1993).

21. Horvath, A. O., & Bedi, R. P. (2002). The alliance. In J. C. Norcross (Ed.), *Psychotherapy relationships that work: Therapist contributions and responsiveness to patients.* New York: Oxford University Press.

22. Shirk, S. R., & Saiz, C. C. (1992). Clinical, empirical, and developmental perspectives on the therapeutic relationship in child psychotherapy. *Development and Psychopathology, 4*, 713–728.

23. Shirk, S. R., & Karver, M. (2003). Prediction of treatment outcome from relationship variables in child and adolescent therapy: A meta-analytic review. *Journal of Consulting and Clinical Psychology, 71*(3), 452–464.

24. Wampold. (2001).

25. Lambert & Barley. (2002).

26. Rhodes, J. (2002). *Stand by me: The risks and rewards of mentoring today's youth.* Cambridge, MA: Harvard University Press.

27. DuBois, D. L., Holloway, B. E., Valentine, J. C., & Cooper, H. (2002). Effectiveness of mentoring programs for youth: A meta-analytic review.

American Journal of Community Psychology, 30(2), 157–197; Grossman, J. B., & Rhodes, J. E. (2002). The test of time: Predictors and effects of duration in youth mentoring programs. *American Journal of Community Psychology, 30,* 199–219.

28. Parra, G. R., DuBois, D. L., Neville, H. A., & Pugh-Lilly, A. O. (2002). Mentoring relationships for youth: Investigation of a process-oriented model. *Journal of Community Psychology, 30*(4), 367–388; DuBois et al. (2002).

29. Liang, B., Tracy, A. J., Taylor, C. A., & Williams, L. M. (2002). Mentoring college-age women: A relational approach. *American Journal of Community Psychology, 30*(2), 271–288; Spencer, R. (2002). *Hanging out and growing strong: A qualitative study of relationships with adults that foster resilience in adolescence.* Unpublished doctoral dissertation, Harvard University.

30. National Research Council and Institute of Medicine. (2002). *Community programs to promote youth development.* Washington, DC: National Academy Press; Rathunde, K. (1996). Family context and talented adolescents' optimal experience in school-related activities. *Journal of Research on Adolescence, 6*(4), 605–628.

31. Vygotsky, L. S. (1978). *Mind in society.* Cambridge, MA: Harvard University Press; Rogoff, B. (1990). *Apprenticeship in thinking: Cognitive development in social context.* New York: Oxford University Press; Rogoff, B. (2003). *The cultural nature of human development.* New York: Oxford University Press.

32. Rogoff. (1990).

33. Darling, N., Hamilton, S. F., & Hames, K. (2003). Relationships outside the family: Unrelated adults. In G. R. Adams & M. D. Berzonsky (Eds.), *Blackwell handbook of adolescence* (pp. 349–370). Cambridge, MA: Blackwell.

34. Rhodes, J. E., Spencer, R., Keller, T. E., Liang, B., & Noam, G. (2004). *A model for the influence of mentoring relationships on youth development.* Manuscript submitted for publication.

35. Spencer, R. (2004). Cavell, T. A., & Hughes, J. N. (2000). Secondary prevention as context for assessing change processes in aggressive children. *Journal of School Psychology, 38,* 199–235.

36. Miller, J. B., & Stiver, I. P. (1997). *The healing connection.* Boston: Beacon Press; Mitchell, S. A. (2000). *Relationality: From attachment to intersubjectivity.* Hillsdale, NJ: Analytic Press; Weissman, M. M., Markowitz, J. C., & Klerman, G. L. (2000). *Comprehensive guide to interpersonal psychotherapy.* New York: Basic Books.

37. Grossman, J. B., & Tierney, J. P. (1998). Does mentoring work? An impact study of the Big Brothers/Big Sisters program. *Evaluation Review, 22,* 403–426; Sipe, C. L. (1996). *Mentoring: A synthesis of the P/PV's research: 1988–1995.* Philadelphia: P/PV; Rhodes, J. E., Reddy, R., Grossman, J. B., & Lee, J. M. (2002). Volunteer mentoring relationships with minority youth: An analysis of same- versus cross-race matches. *Journal of Applied Social Psychology, 32*(10), 2114–2133.

38. Grossman & Rhodes. (2002).

39. Sue, D. W., & Sue, D. (2003). *Counseling the culturally diverse: Theory and practice* (4th ed.). New York: Wiley.

40. Sarason, B. R., & Sarason, I. G. (2001). Ongoing aspects of relationships

and health outcomes: Social support, social control, companionship, and relationship meaning. In J. Harvey & A. Wenzel (Eds.), *Close romantic relationships: Maintenance and enhancement* (pp. 277–298). Mahwah, NJ: Erlbaum.

41. Rook, K. S. (1995). Support, companionship, and control in older adults' social networks: Implications for well-being. In J. F. Nussbaum & J. Coupland (Eds.), *Handbook of communication and aging research* (pp. 437–463). Mahwah, NJ: Erlbaum.

42. Morrow, K. V., & Styles, M. B. (1995). *Building relationships with youth in program settings: A study of Big Brothers/Big Sisters.* Philadelphia: Public/Private Ventures; Spencer, R., Jordan, J. V., & Sazama, J. (in press). Growth-promoting relationships between youth and adults: A focus group study. *Families in Society.*

RENEÉ SPENCER *is an assistant professor at the Boston University School of Social Work.*

Positive teacher-student relationships are seen through a variety of psychological models.

4

The role of teacher relationships in the lives of students

Katia Fredriksen, Jean Rhodes

AS ALL PARENTS KNOW, children's relationships with their teachers can be a crucially important influence, affecting students' connection to school, motivation, academic performance, and psychosocial well-being. Students spend a great deal of time at school, and the classroom is the source of many of their interpersonal relationships and activities. Although children's social adjustment to school was initially examined primarily through relationships with classroom peers, research increasingly has highlighted the significance of student-teacher relationships.[1]

Academic achievement

Relationships with teachers may have an impact on students' learning and academic achievement. Children with better social skills may be more adept at interacting in positive ways with teachers and peers, and teachers may interpret positive interactions as reflecting not only social competence but also intellectual competence. In addition, children who are motivated to seek approval from their teachers may employ achievement-related behaviors to meet this

NEW DIRECTIONS FOR YOUTH DEVELOPMENT, NO. 103, FALL 2004 © WILEY PERIODICALS, INC.

goal. Finally, supportive relationships with teachers may augment students' motivation to learn and actively participate in subject domains that have traditionally held little interest for them. Increased participation may result in changes in attitude regarding the subject domain as students experience increased efficacy, interest, and perceived utility.[2]

Psychological adjustment

While most work to date has focused on academic outcomes, there is growing evidence that perceptions of support from teachers also affect psychological adjustment. In a preschool population, researchers found that secure attachment with a teacher partially compensated for insecure child-mother attachment relationships, predicting teacher-rated social competence and prosocial behavior. In an elementary school population, students who reported more positive bonds with their teachers obtained higher scores on self- and teacher-reported social and emotional adjustment outcomes. In addition, elementary school children appear to make judgments about their classmates based on perceptions of how the target child interacts with and is perceived by the teacher, which has implications for peer acceptance and rejection.[3]

Teacher support also appears to have an impact on psychological adjustment in older students. Students who attended middle schools that deliberately sought to enhance teacher-student relationships tended to have fewer adjustment difficulties during the transition. Indeed, changes in perceptions of teacher support predicted changes in both self-esteem and depression among middle school students, such that students who perceived increasing teacher support showed corresponding decreases in depressive symptoms and increases in self-esteem, while students who perceived decreasing teacher support showed increased depressive symptoms and decreased self-esteem. Other researchers have emphasized the impact of positive teacher relationships on students' social development, with this support serving a regulatory function in children's and adolescents' development of not only academic and behavioral skills but also emotional skills. These findings suggest that teacher support can help to buffer some of the stress associated with middle school, offsetting the risk for adjustment difficulties.[4]

Factors contributing to the quality of student-teacher relationships

Researchers have identified a number of factors that contribute to the quality of student-teacher relationships. The development of these relationships is a dynamic process that is built on the beliefs, values, and skills of both participants. Elementary school students who believe that they are good at interacting with their teachers are more likely to report a warm student-teacher relationship and to report turning to their teacher when they need emotional or academic support, as well as modeling themselves after their teacher. Students who exhibit problem behaviors, including inattention, internalizing, and disruptive and aggressive behaviors, are likely to have negative relationships with their teachers that may be critical and punishing, and characterized by conflict and a lack of warmth. In addition, students who experience greater dissatisfaction with the school environment, or who are reluctant to use adults as a source of support or to invest in relationships with adults, are likely to experience less supportive relationships with their teachers.[5]

Teacher characteristics also play an important role in the formation of close ties with students. Researchers have linked teachers' attachment histories with their primary caregiver with the quality of student-teacher relationships. Elementary teachers' levels of stress and negative affect predicted the number of students with whom teachers had negative relationships. Teachers who are stressed may be more likely to display inappropriate negative affect, such as anger and hostility, thereby creating an adversarial stance with students. Teachers' images of themselves as educators, as well as their beliefs about their efficacy in the classroom and their expectations for students, also appear to influence the ways in which they interact with students, as do their gender, experience, socioeconomic status, education, and ethnicity.[6]

Theoretical models

Researchers have presented a number of models that have somewhat different ways of framing positive student-teacher relationships and the role students and teachers play in forming these. Researchers who view student-teacher relationships through an attachment lens conceptualize them as extensions of the parent-child relationship. From an attachment perspective, warm, supportive, caring relationships characterized by open communication, trust, involvement, and responsiveness are necessary to help children develop behavioral, social, cognitive, and emotional skills.[7] Good student-teacher relationships are characterized by low levels of conflict and high levels of closeness, supporting children's motivation to explore as well as their growing ability to regulate social, emotional, and cognitive skills. Children use their relational models concerning the nature of social relationships and their social world, including conceptions of emotional closeness, conflict, and dependency, to shape interpretations of classroom interactions. Children who have experienced insecurity with primary attachment figures are likely to be ambivalent toward exploration and intimacy experiences, while children who have formed secure attachments with primary caretakers are likely to have the skills to engage more adaptively in these sorts of experiences.

Teachers also play a role in shaping relationships through the emotional quality of their interactions with children, as well as their responsiveness in terms of frequency and consistency to children's needs. They can be particularly important to early adolescents, who are often undergoing profound shifts in their sense of self and are struggling to negotiate changing relationships with their parents and peers. Since teachers have the advantage of standing outside these struggles, they can provide a safe context for support and guidance, while transmitting adult values, advice, and perspectives.[8]

Motivation researchers tend to concentrate on the role that teachers play as effective instructors, citing evidence that students rely not only on the structure and support that teachers can provide but also on teachers' ability to help them feel successful academically.[9] Teachers' expectations, beliefs, and behaviors are thought to shape the quality of their relationships with students. For example, the extent to which teachers are able to balance the need for structure within the classroom with students' need for autonomy predicts students' internalization of responsibility for their learning and motivation to do well, as well as feelings of competence. Research suggests that by creating an environment that encourages feelings of belonging and support, teachers can simultaneously meet the academic and social needs of students.

Sociocultural perspectives on student-teacher relationships introduce yet another way of assessing their quality and impact, focusing on the nested structures associated with these relationships, which are embedded within classrooms, which in turn are embedded within schools, which in turn are embedded with an academic culture. Ecological studies have demonstrated the reciprocal nature of student-teacher relationships and the ways in which classrooms, schools, communities, and other systems interact to affect the quality of these relationships. For example, teachers provide a more positive emotional climate in the classroom and have more frequent interactions with specific students when class size is lower. In addition, when students perceive the school climate as caring, they tend to view their relationships with teachers more positively. Research on the classroom system shows that students' relationships with peers and with the school may have an impact on their relationships with teachers; for example, the extent to which peer norms correspond to teacher and academic norms is likely to influence the quality of student-teacher relationships. In addition, students' perceptions of teachers' relationships with other students in the classroom may influence their own relationship with the teacher.[10]

Developmental systems theory also views student-teacher relationships in the context of a number of systems.[11] The developing child, a system in and of himself or herself, functions in the context of proximal (for example, temperament) and more distal (for example, student-teacher relationships) systems. Within the school setting, interactions take place within and across levels, as teachers are influenced by their beliefs about a particular child as well as by their training and the school in which they work, and these interactions are reciprocal and bidirectional. The child's competence springs from both the child's characteristics, such as attention and cognition, and the child's relations and interactions in the context of the classroom. Relationships between children and adults are largely responsible for developmental change, and relationships with teachers form developmental stepping-stones on which students' later school experiences build.

The role of schools

Student-teacher relationships deeply influence students' academic and psychosocial functioning. Although different models vary in their explanation of these effects, none denies their existence. As demonstrated, evidence suggests that student-teacher relationships remain important throughout students' academic careers, with research spanning from preschool to high school. However, close and confiding student-teacher relationships appear to be more the exception than the rule. Students may develop one or two important ties with certain teachers over the course of their schooling, but they do not perceive their typical teacher relationships as particularly close or meaningful.[12]

Given the way schools are structured, this is not surprising. The same teachers who are being asked to provide more personalized support are simultaneously being saddled with additional obligations. A growing emphasis on high-stakes standardized testing has given rise to dense curricular demands that have constrained teachers and left little room for the sorts of conversations and activities that typically draw them closer to their students. Larger student-teacher ratios have left each young person with a smaller piece of the teacher's attention. Sadly, many adults who were initially drawn to the teaching profession out of a desire to establish meaningful connections with their students have become increasingly disillusioned by the structural impediments to relationships in schools. Supportive bonds become even less practical as students move into middle and high school and no longer have a primary teacher with whom they spend most of the day. Rather than presenting impediments, schools should increase the likelihood of teacher-student bonds.

The supportive potential of teachers has not gone entirely unnoticed among school reformers, however, and they recommend a broad array of efforts to capitalize on it. A major challenge for schools will be to create settings that can increase and facilitate teachers' and other staff members' caring potential, while maintaining academic rigor and teacher autonomy. In addition to making teacher salaries more competitive (the starting salaries of New York City teachers hover around $30,000 per year) and establishing a corps of highly qualified and high-quality teachers, we should evaluate school policies in terms of their effects on student-teacher relationships.

There is unequivocal evidence that lowered student-teacher ratios are associated with improved student achievement and competence, and this is a straightforward means of improving teacher-student interactions. Similarly, policies that ensure more contact and continuity with teachers, such as homerooms, advising, and multiyear teacher assignments, might provide students with support for learning and development through relationships. Resources should be deployed that enhance student-teacher fit such that the student feels supported and the teacher feels effective.

Interventions at the school climate level can affect student-teacher contact and quality through restructuring of time and scheduling, allocation of space and teaching resources, placement policies, and work related to school values, cultural issues, and staff support and involvement in decision making. Such programs, involving changes at the classroom level, such as the Child Development Project, or within specific student-teacher interactions, such as the Students, Teachers, and Relationship Support (STARS) system, should be more widely implemented, so that children and adolescents can reap the many benefits associated with positive student-teacher relationships.[13]

Notes

1. Barber, B. K., & Olsen, J. A. (2004). Assessing the transitions to middle and high school. *Journal of Adolescent Research 19*(1), 3–30; Birch, S. H., & Ladd, G. W. (1997). The teacher-child relationship and children's early school adjustment. *Journal of School Psychology, 35*(1), 61–79; Pianta, R. C., Stuhlman, M., & Hamre, B. (2002). How schools can do better: Fostering stronger connections between teachers and students. In J. E. Rhodes (Ed.), *A critical view of youth mentoring* (pp. 91–107). San Francisco: Jossey-Bass.

2. Brophy, K., & Hancock, S. (1985). Adult-child interaction in an integrated preschool programme: Implications for teacher training. *Early Child Development and Care, 22*(4), 275–294; Ford, M. E. (1982). Social cognition and social competence in adolescence. *Developmental Psychology, 18*, 323–340; Urdan, T., & Maehr, M. (1995). Beyond a two-goal theory of motivation and achievement: A case for social goals. *Review of Educational Research, 65*, 213–243.

3. Colarossi, L. G., & Eccles, J. S. (2003). Differential effects of support providers on adolescents' mental health. *Social Work Research, 27*(1), 19–30; Hoge, D. R., Smit, E. K., & Hanson, S. L. (1990). School experiences predicting changes in self-esteem of sixth- and seventh-grade students. *Journal of Educational Psychology, 82*(1), 117–127; Hughes, J. N., Cavell, T. A., & Jackson, T. (1999). Influence of teacher-student relationship on childhood conduct problems: A prospective study. *Journal of Clinical Child Psychology, 38*, 173–184; Mitchell-Copeland, J., Denham, S. A., & DeMulder, E. K. (1997). Q-sort assessment of child-teacher attachment relationships and social competence in the preschool. *Early Education and Development, 8*(1), 27–39; Murray, C., & Greenberg, M. T. (2001). Relationships with teachers and bonds with school: Social emotional adjustment correlates for children with and without disabilities. *Psychology in the Schools, 38*(1), 25–41.

4. Davis, H. A. (2003). Conceptualizing the role and influence of student-teacher relationships on children's social and cognitive development. *Educational Psychologist, 38*(4), 207–234; Midgley, C., & Edelin, K. C. (1998). Middle school reform and early adolescent well-being: The good news and the bad. *Educational Psychologist, 33*(4), 195–206; Pianta, R. C. (1999). *Enhancing relationships between children and teachers.* Washington, DC: American Psychological Association; Pianta, Stuhlman, & Hamre. (2002).

5. Coie, J. D., & Koeppl, G. K. (1990). Adapting intervention to the problems of aggressive and disruptive children. In S. R. Asher & J. D. Coie (Eds.), *Peer rejection in childhood* (pp. 309–337). Cambridge: Cambridge University Press; Davis, H. A. (2001). The quality and impact of relationships between

elementary school students and teachers. *Contemporary Educational Psychology*, *26*, 431–453; Mitchell-Copeland, Denham, & DeMulder. (1997); Pianta, R. C., & Nimetz, S. L. (1991). Relationships between children and teachers: Associations with classroom and home behavior. *Journal of Applied Development Psychology*, *12*, 379–393; Itskowitz, R., Navon, R., & Strauss, H. (1988). Teachers' accuracy in evaluating students' self-image: Effects of perceived closeness. *Journal of Educational Psychology*, *80*, 337–341.

   6. Kesner, J. (2000). Teacher characteristics and the quality of child-teacher relationships. *Journal of School Psychology*, *28*(2), 133–149; Pianta, R. C., Hamre, B., & Stuhlman, M. (2003). Relationships between teachers and children. In W. M. Reynolds & G. E. Miller (Eds.), *Handbook of psychology: educational psychology* (Vol. 7, pp. 199–234). New York: Wiley; Yoon, J. S. (2002). Teacher characteristics as predictors of teacher-student relationships: Stress, negative affect, and self-efficacy. *Social Behavior and Personality*, *30*(5), 485–494.

   7. Baker, J. A., & Bridger, R. (1997). Schools as caring communities: A relational approach to school reform. *School Psychology Review*, *26*(4), 586–602; Bowlby, J. (1982). *Attachment and loss*. New York: Basic Books; Murray, C., & Greenberg, M. T. (2000). Children's relationships with teachers and bonds with school: An investigation of patterns and correlates in middle childhood. *Journal of School Psychology*, *38*, 423–445.

   8. Davis (2003); Lynch, M., & Cicchetti, D. (1992). Maltreated children's reports of relatedness to their teachers. In R. C. Pianta (Ed.), *Beyond the parent: The role of other adults in children's lives* (pp. 81–107). San Francisco: Jossey-Bass; Lynch, M., & Cicchetti, D. (1997). Children's relationships with adults and peers: An examination of elementary and junior high school students. *Journal of School Psychology*, *35*, 87–100; Resnick, M. D., Bearman, P. S., Blum, R. W., Bauman, K. E., Harris, K. M., Jones, J., Tabor, J., Beuhring, T., Sieving, R. E., Shew, M., Ireland, M., Bearinger, L. H., & Udry, J. R. (1998). Protecting adolescents from harm: Finding from the national longitudinal study of adolescent health. In R. E. Muuss & H. D. Porton (Eds.), *Adolescent behavior and society: A book of readings*. New York: McGraw-Hill; Rhodes, J. E., Grossman, J. B., & Resch, N. R. (2000). Agents of change: Pathways through which mentoring relationships influence adolescents' academic adjustment. *Child Development*, *71*, 1662–1671.

   9. Davis, H. A. (2001). The quality and impact of relationships between elementary school students and teachers. *Contemporary Educational Psychology*, *26*, 431–453; Davis (2003).

   10. Battistich, V., Solomon, D., Watson, M., & Schaps, E. (1997). Caring school communities. *Educational Psychologist*, *32*(3), 137–151; NICHD Early Child Care Research Network. (2001, April). *Observations in first-grade classrooms: The other side of school readiness*. Paper presented at the biennial meeting of the Society for Research in Child Development, Minneapolis, MN.

   11. Pianta, Hamre, & Stuhlman (2003).

   12. Lempers, J. D., & Clark-Lempers, D. S. (1992). Young, middle, and late adolescents' comparisons of the functional importance of five significant relationships. *Journal of Youth and Adolescence*, *21*(1), 53–96.

   13. According to Pianta, Stuhlman, and Hamre (2002), the Child Development Project is designed to promote social and moral development, a sense of

community, and caring for students. This program has primarily been implemented in elementary schools, with interventions at both the classroom and school levels. In contrast, the Students, Teachers, and Relationship Support (STARS) system is designed to help the teacher improve his or her relationship with a particular student. The program uses a supportive relationship with a consultant to target the teacher's representation of his or her relationship with the student as well as the teacher's behavior toward the student.

KATIA FREDRIKSEN *is a doctoral candidate in the clinical psychology program at the University of Massachusetts Boston.*

JEAN RHODES *is professor of psychology at the University of Massachusetts Boston, a clinical and community psychologist, and a fellow of the American Psychological Association.*

Personal mentoring connections between teachers and students in high school are unique components of the developmental process and carry great potential for community-building at school.

5

Learning relationships: Teacher-student connections, learning, and identity in high school

Beth Bernstein-Yamashiro

"SHE WAS MY English teacher in ninth grade and we had to talk about ourselves and write about it . . . she didn't just read our stories that were about us and just grade them and give them back to us. She would talk to us about 'em. If there was something that she thought needed to be talked about individually she would talk to you. Or if you wanted to talk about it, you could talk to her. And she would go out of her time to do it and she wouldn't just hand the paper back and say, 'It wasn't written right.' Even if the writing wasn't good, she would still discuss it." In this display of encouragement, caring, and challenge from his teacher, Alex, a tenth-grade student, experiences the excitement of learning from a teacher who nurtures both his ability to write and learn, as well as his self-expression as a developing adolescent. Curriculum is a medium through which intellectual curiosity and personal development can be shared; the relationship between student and teacher provides a foundation on which deeply satisfying learning

NEW DIRECTIONS FOR YOUTH DEVELOPMENT, NO. 103, FALL 2004 © WILEY PERIODICALS, INC.

can be built. In this learning relationship, Alex and his teacher work together to create shared understandings in an atmosphere of learning and growth.

Although most educators acknowledge that teaching and learning are highly interpersonal activities, the tenor of teacher-student relationships is an often-overlooked area of study or of policy attention. Persistent dropout and school failure, as well as the rash of school violence over the past decade, have caused many educators to examine what adults might do to connect better with young people in their schools and communities. The study on which this chapter is based reveals that relationships—personal mentoring connections between teachers and students in high school—represent powerful and creative efforts to cross the widening chasm between adults and teenagers. These relationships are not simply special additions for those who engage in them. Rather, they constitute learning opportunities of their own, unique components of the developmental process, and a potential for community-building at school.

Educational policy tends to consider only those variables over which policymakers believe they have some control. Issues like opportunities for personal interaction, students' affective experiences of learning, or teachers' emotional health seem overly serendipitous and tangential to academic achievement, and so they are not on the policy table. Nonetheless, studies consistently cite a failure to connect with an adult as a major variable in dropout.[1] A few recent studies have begun to document the importance of positive relationships between teachers and students in student achievement or effective classrooms.[2] Data from my study portray relationships as key ingredients in successful teaching and learning. Students, as well as teachers, are constantly negotiating their identities and searching for personal validation in relationships at school. Learning relationships challenge educators to synthesize these complex processes so that they become integral to definitions of pedagogy. As teachers and administrators think about what they want students to know and be able to do, they must consider who students will become and how their relationships with them will contribute to their emerging identities as both human beings and thoughtful intellectuals.

The data gathered for this study were collected over a semester at a high school with eighteen hundred students located in a small, urban, ethnically diverse, working- to middle-class neighborhood of a large metropolis in the West. I conducted ninety-one one-hour interviews, including focus groups and individual interviews, with 27 teachers and 117 students in tenth through twelfth grades. Participants volunteered based on their assertions that they had experienced close, personal teacher-student relationships. Students ranged from high achievers to at-risk students. I interviewed both sides of these relationships in order to gain a multidimensional perspective. In focus group interviews, participants were able to search together for ways to describe and categorize their perspectives. In individual follow-up interviews, I explored layers of meaning within the framework of relationship building.

Participants defined teacher-student relationships as those connections that emerge when students initiate conversations with teachers during or after class, surrounding classwork, or their outside lives.[3] In describing their close relationships with teachers, participants struggled for appropriate words. "It's like a friend," one sophomore offered, "but like an older friend," "Like a close uncle," explained one senior, "He's my stand-in dad," said another. "Teacher-friend" implied that the two roles operated in tandem. These students' struggles with language suggest that the relationships are distinct; they are similar to but not completely like any other connections they have with peers or family members. Teachers spend their days with teenagers but are themselves adults, with wisdom to tap into and experience to share. They do not enjoy parental authority, but they do have a greater sense of right and wrong than do peers. The relationships described comprise a spectrum, from a student feeling close to a teacher who patiently explained math concepts, to a teacher who considered herself a student's "on-site mom."

This chapter addresses how teacher-student relationships bear on students' learning experiences and their concurrent efforts to form their emerging identities. Despite the fact that many secondary educators are not convinced that forming relationships with students has much to do with learning, I argue here that teachers cannot attempt to cultivate teenagers' intellects while leaving behind their emotional development. It is in recognizing and respecting the inextricable link between the two that teachers can make considerable academic impact.

Fear and coping in class

While the size and schedules of most public schools assume teenagers to be less in need of coddling than preadolescents, many students described high degrees of classroom anxiety due not only to their fears of peer judgment but from their perceptions of many teachers as unapproachable, impatient, or hostile. Students are extremely nervous about understanding material and being able to do their work. Consistently, they depicted the rigid and impersonal demeanors of most of their teachers as the context in which they situated the one or two close relationships they had:

There are classes where the attitude that the teacher gives us and the way the teacher doesn't treat us as though they like us, as though we're just here for the learning, no fun involved at all, it's just such a bad environment. You're so upset with the teacher, you can't even sit there and learn [Daisha, grade 12].

Students described their emotional responses to these teachers as governing much of their academic behavior. They often did not seek help learning material from teachers who seemed threatening,[4] and they did not take intellectual risks in uncomfortable settings.

Students need to feel confident enough to access academic support, discuss grades, and make up missed assignments. In an unfortunate misinterpretation, many teachers read students' not asking for help as a sign that students do not want to learn. In fact, students are disappointed and hurt when teachers do not fully explain material:

If half the class gets it and some of the class doesn't, he'll just keep going anyway. He's gotta make sure the whole class understands it no matter what. . . . The teacher and her students are supposed to be like friends. If half the class is getting an F, I don't think the teacher's doing her job. She shouldn't just keep moving. She should go back so the kids can get good grades. No matter how long it takes [Jason, grade 10].

Many students in this study believed that most teachers did not care about students' success. Therefore, teachers who helped students learn material were seen as extending friendship and validating students as people:

I think the most important thing is if a teacher takes time to explain things to you if you don't understand. 'Cause that makes you feel that you're important enough for them that they would actually take some of their own time for you. Even if it's after school . . . if it's their own time, then that's *me*, it's just me and them, so I guess that means that I'm important enough to them that they'd actually want to help me during their own time [Carrie, grade 10].

I'd be like, "I'm ready for you to help me out." And he'd help me with like three problems, and maybe I would have gotten one, but then there's still another whole page of twenty problems that are *different*, that I didn't understand. Mr. Pippen was the kind of teacher, he'd help you with all twenty problems, and he would never even sigh. He would sit down right next to me and we'd have *my* calculator and *my* pen and he'd just help, like kind of guide me through it [Laurie, grade 11].

Despite the fact that teachers' jobs ordinarily require staying after school to help students or call parents, most students interpret this help as a profound sign of care. Teachers who convey that they care about students' learning or patiently explain material alleviate the anxieties that preclude student performance.

While certain teachers claim that connecting with students is daunting or inappropriate, most students felt that relationships did not have to extend beyond the classroom or be particularly intense; rather, any attempt by teachers to break the ice or express caring made an enormous difference to students' interest, confidence, and motivation. Callie, a senior, explained, "It's simple . . . you have to be good with people to get things across. Even with your math teacher." Added Regina, another senior, "I'm just talking about the occasional, 'How ya doing? Everything going all right?' or 'That was a really good essay you wrote.'" Bruce Klein, a social studies teacher, concurred: "You call them by name, you make eye contact. These are things you do as a valid person, a person who cares about others."

Teachers who participated in this study believed that warm relationships were instrumental to effective pedagogy:

I try to make the classroom a safe and comfortable place for them to be, and I want them to know when they come in my room, I'm not going to yell at them. I never yell at kids. I'm not going to make them feel bad. I'm not going to allow anyone else in the room to make them feel bad. And I feel like that's really my job as a teacher before anything else, to let kids know that they are welcome, that they have a right to be there, and dress the way they want, and do their own thing and be themselves. I see that as my first job. Everything else comes second [Eileen, computer teacher].

Students asserted that the experience of learning material is rarely separated from how they feel while they learn and how they feel about the person from whom they learn. This dramatic intertwining demands that educators reimagine definitions of pedagogy and cognition, especially as they relate to motivation. Teacher-student relationships are integral to pedagogy—as important as a teacher's syllabus, classroom activities, or written feedback.

Consent to learn

Students use schoolwork and academic behavior to communicate many messages to teachers. If teachers treat students in a disrespectful or humiliating manner, student participants claimed they would not do that teacher's work or pay attention in class, as that teacher's overall judgment was in question. As one sophomore explained, "Those teachers who have attitudes, and who aren't really there for you, you're like, 'Why do I even do this work? Why would I bother?'" Lee, a history teacher, articulated the same phenomenon from her perspective:

I think that's really the only way you can be effective as a teacher. Because if it's, "Here's the history and learn it and take a test," if they don't connect with you, those kids are not going to learn anything from you. You're just a voice at the front of the classroom, and they don't care about you when they know you don't care about them.

Conversely, teachers' encouragement can inspire students to make efforts in class and indicates to students that they are valued as people and respected intellectually.[5] While they may be able to elicit such support from parents, the objective confirmation of a teacher provides students unique inspiration to perform:

Mr. Barrington knew that I could do it but that I didn't push myself. . . . He was telling me, "Come in during lunch if you need help." And I used to come in, and I passed that class with a B. It's weird because all my teachers, they see that "She's a person who wants to do her work, she has the potential, but she doesn't do it." I need motivation from people, like "You can do it, you can do it" [Trina, grade 11].

Learning relationships are complex and two-sided. Teachers give students support and advice, provide academic help, and create classroom community. Students use academic behavior on homework, participation, positive behavior, and test performance to communicate their respect and hold up their sides of the friendships:

If you get to know a teacher, you get on a personal basis. You don't want to let that teacher down, so you work harder to keep your grades up [Jon, grade 12].

I got to the point where it was expected out of me, not just because I had done well in class, but because I felt like I owed it to her, as friends. Just like if you're on a team with someone—I felt that I owed it to her in a sense that she was a good teacher and that I wanted to show her that I was getting taught and I wasn't wasting my time in her class [Megan, grade 10].

Students' efforts in school are greatly dependent on their feelings of care, encouragement, and investment from their teachers. They are deliberate in their decisions to work or withhold academic effort, to participate or misbehave. Teachers' failure to understand students' academic behavior can lead to negative classroom cycles. These data reveal the value of listening to students to appreciate why it is they might refuse to learn.

Creating a human identity at school

High school is a place where students are working out who they are and who they want to become. Forming an identity is not only a task of adolescence;[6] it is a vital aspect of student life. Relationships with teachers are important contexts for students' efforts to understand themselves; they can provide personal validation and enable necessary reflection. As students search to understand self and self-in-relation-to-others, they look to teachers for confirmation that they are "good people," that they can learn if taught well, and that they are unique individuals with outside lives and challenges. The relationships are venues wherein students can counteract negative assumptions about teenagers, test out ideas, and be seen for who they are.

For participants, a major aspect of their efforts to establish their identities involved rejecting prescribed institutional roles. Students consistently described a distinction between "teachers who teach" and "teachers who are people." Their definitions underscore how important it is to them that teachers break through these roles and be reachable human beings:

I think that respect starts when the teacher stops looking at you like your stereotype, sees you as a person that has potential to do well in your class and just sees you as a person. Just a normal person that they can talk to. Just a person in the world, not just a student that they have to help or teach [Lisa, grade 11].

In addition to finding many of their teachers burned out, unfulfilled, and uncaring, these teachers were seen as disregarding students' own humanity. It seemed that students wanted teachers to be "people" so that students would feel that they too could be human. The valued teachers saw students as "people" and not just "students," a role students found limiting and demeaning:

He jokes around. He treats you like a person, not like a student. There's teachers who treat you like they're superior, and you're there under their command and you must listen to them. Mr. Cameron teaches you but does it in a way that's just like a friend showing you something [Adelina, grade 10].

When a teacher knows your name and knows who you are, it's uplifting because you're not just a face in the class. You're a person who they respect. They don't just walk by and say, "Hello student in the first row" [Keith, grade 12].

As they seek to establish their identities, students need teachers to accept them for their likes and interests. Thus, they felt judged by teachers who appeared prejudiced against students because of their identification with popular culture:

I think some teachers see themselves as completely different from the students. They see that kids are into their own kind of music and their own kind of stuff. And they don't want to have anything to do with that. . . . So like some teachers think, "all rap [music] is bad." So if students listen to it, they must be bad too [Alex, grade 10].

To counteract such prejudice, certain students initiated teacher-student relationships. Emily, a goth-clothed, facially pierced sophomore explained:

I get to know the teachers because of the way I look. I don't want them to stereotype me by like not giving me an answer to a question just because of the way I look, so I want them to know me on a level like, "Hey I'm a nice person, I have honors grades."

While trying to develop as young adults, students reject the authority that teachers assert because of position, age, or emotional distance. Through their schoolwork, their own initiation of relationships with teachers, and their refusal to respect teachers who do not treat them as valued individuals, students communicate deep messages to the adult world about who they want to be and how they want to learn. Teachers who understand that students want to be validated as "people" and not processed as "students," who create safe atmospheres for intellectual risk, and who express their own personalities to students understand the complexities that determine many students' dispositions to learn.

Growing and learning in relationships

Despite the prevalent belief that teens do not respect or want to know adults,[7] data in my study indicate that it is *students* who feel disconnected and desire strong personal relationships with adults. Many students noted that teenage life today is separate from adult life and completely unlike the adolescences that teachers experienced. Students today find they have reduced outside community support, limited access to extended families, and little time to spend with parents.[8] They find that relationships with teachers can help fill these gaps in support. Students want teachers to help them work out problems without judging their behavior. Within these relationships, they create a familial atmosphere within large schools and empower teachers to inhabit roles as supportive advisers. Finally, the relationships themselves have a developmental aspect: as students move from the beginning of high school to the end and develop into young adults, their needs in and perspectives on relationships change. Their experiences within relationships enable them to learn and grow.

In relationships with their "adult friends," students learn critical relationship skills that are noted characteristics of resilient children.[9] They learn how to express their needs and receive care from a nonfamilial adult:

It's kind of like an adult friendship. They have that adult standpoint where they can see it from the point of view of an adult, but also see it as a friend, and someone who understands what you're going through. . . . They're not just like kidding around conversations too . . . you can actually talk with a person on the same kind of level and that's what makes you feel really good [Megan, grade 10].

Students often do not feel comfortable seeking advice from family members for fear of punishment or judgment. They therefore look to teachers to fulfill a parental but uninvolved role. Solving problems appeared vital to students' confidence; teachers could help them learn the skills they needed to work things out on their own:

Your parents are responsible for you and they care for you and they can punish you. A teacher can't punish you. They don't have that authority. All they can do is listen to you and try to help you with your problem. If you get drunk at a party, they can't punish you. You're not their child. So all they can do is advise you [Kathy, grade 11].

Not only are teachers objective elders, they are able to bring a broader ethical understanding to their interactions with students that students cannot find with peers:

Ms. Jamison will play that mother role and tell me, "You know, this is right and wrong." And if she notices that I do something wrong, she will be like, "Have you looked at it this way?" She won't tell me I'm wrong; she will say, "Well, look at it this way." And she makes me see the bad side of it [Joaquín, grade 12].

Students not only received help working out problems; they were able to learn about the world they were about to enter:

When you talk to people who are actually adults and have actually lived, you know how to use your people skills more. And it teaches you how to interact with people outside of school . . . it gives you people skills about people who have already grown and know the world [Christina, grade 12].

A few students offered that if teachers wanted to be more effective and human with their students, they needed to acknowledge problems students face in their outside lives:

Some adults do not understand that you go through things when you're a teenager. Some teachers are just like, "Well that's your problem, don't bring it to school." Other teachers will understand and try to help you out with it [Shamika, grade 12].

Teachers should be to the point where a student can go up to them when they're having problems or something. Sometimes students come into class, they're having stuff at home and the teachers don't want to ask, "What's happening?" or, "Talk to me, tell me why you're acting like this?" [Luis, grade 10].

Teacher-student relationships tend to develop concurrently with students' maturation. As sophomores, students focus heavily on understanding curriculum and are less willing to seek personal advice and support; as seniors look toward their futures, they need teachers to help them understand the world they are about to enter. Two seniors explain:

As you reach senior year, the work becomes kind of secondary to your personal relationships. 'Cause you're focusing on what's gonna happen in the real world. And the best way to get that started is to have a relationship with adults that you're around. When teachers are dealing with a sophomore, they're dealing with a person who still doesn't know who they are. A sophomore just sees the teacher as giving work. Teachers treat seniors more as adults [Keith, grade 12].

When you're a sophomore, you still kind of care about academics. I'm not saying seniors don't. But I care more about how people are, why they do what they do [Joaquín, grade 12].

In friendships with teachers, students begin to interact with adults and model adult behavior as they prepare themselves for life after school. While deeply involved in trying to understand themselves, students learned in their teacher-student relationships what they could give to a relationship and what they wanted from it, and they deeply valued the degree of equality that they felt they achieved in such a relationship by senior year.

Several teacher participants also described their teaching roles to include being "adult friends" to students. Most teachers who felt this way were motivated by a moral sense that they could not ignore students' needs or pretend that school curricula were the central aspect of students' lives:

I think they're looking for someone who can give meaning to not only why they're here in an academic sense, but to help show them socially how their lives connect with each other. School is more than academics. It's a social organization that can provide a lot of structured meaning for things later on in life. How is it that you effectively deal with people? I think they look at teachers as guidance people to get them through a lot of different things [Jim, science teacher].

Certainly when kids have got rough or abusive situations at home, with the drama students I think I'm certainly the one they're most likely to talk to—just those great talks that kids need to have with adults . . . about where life goes and what happens in the world [Jake, drama teacher].

The teachers who reached out to students were more than simply empathetic. They believed that teaching requires mentoring. And while talking with students outside class proved draining for some teachers, all of those who chose to perform these functions saw important learning taking place in these relationships.

Conclusions and implications

In discussions over achievement, policy tends to dichotomize academic from affective realms. Debates center on whether feelings or emotions are issues with which schools should be concerned. But schools deal daily with socioemotional issues—when students drop out, when they are absent, when they act out, and when they fail. Whether adults choose to acknowledge it, students experience emotional responses to teachers' behavior and interpret messages from the adults around them for signs of validation or rejection. For students, being able to learn depends on their feeling known, cared for, and respected as emerging young adults.

Most large public school structures assume a particular conception of how adolescence ought to proceed: that students should handle their emotional lives on their own time. Students in this study argued that they do not and cannot separate their emotions from their intellects. School is a place where adolescent identity is constantly forming and changing. It happens in hallways, in classrooms, on playing fields, and with teachers, friends, and coaches. Schools do not need to create life skills classes to contribute to students' emerging identities. But by ignoring students' needs for adult support and wisdom and not acknowledging the complex interaction of affect and intellect, schools fail to maximize students' growth and teachers' understanding.

Sizer contends, "Good schools are thoughtful places. The people in them are known. The units are small enough to be coherent communities of friends."[10] In large, alienating schools, students can feel dehumanized. Many students as well as teachers in this study claimed that there was never enough time to talk about academic material outside class, discuss other issues, or simply get to know one another as individuals. Increasingly, there are many examples of schools and school districts that have chosen to focus on personalization as a means to improved academic achievement.[11] They are redesigning large high schools in an effort to limit student-teacher ratios and create positive relationships. These schools and the adults within them go beyond recognizing that relationships between teachers and students are means to important ends of learning. They agree that the relationships are critical to establishing school norms of community, care, and responsibility to society. Adults in such schools accept personalization as an underlying value communicated in school mission, structure, and classroom pedagogy.

One student in this study argued that a disposition to relate well with students could not be taught, "It's more of an art," he claimed. "You can't really teach it." Nonetheless, relating well with adolescents, having patience, or understanding how students interpret difficult material cannot be characterized as fortuitous personality traits. Rather, preservice education and teacher professional development must help teachers find ways to centralize these and other similar findings. Students state that simply greeting them at the door, knowing their names, asking them questions about their activities, or the occasional "hello," make them feel more welcomed in class and disposed to learn. Others noted that individual help with material alleviated their intellectual anxieties and propelled them to succeed. Teacher educators need not advocate that teachers love students or become more sensitive individuals; rather, the complexities of adolescent development can be incorporated into discussions about effective pedagogy. School administrators who supervise teachers can easily include classroom atmosphere as a point of evaluation and discuss strategies for effective relationships. Staying after school to help students deal with material is a job requirement in almost every school district, but many teachers do not stay or do not invite students into their classroom for help. Schools can structure out-of-class assistance without overwhelming teachers who already feel the strain of heavy student loads or the pressures of standardized testing. Finally, school or district goals can reflect a disposition toward creating caring intellectual communities. If educators believe the central task to be increasing student achievement, then they must continually search to understand what students really need in order to learn.

Teachers and students in this study revealed that in their experiences of creating and sustaining positive teacher-student relationships, they learned about themselves, learned important skills of relating to and caring about others, and creatively infused a personal dimension into the educational encounter. These relationships reveal that while school is indeed intended to be about learning, learning itself proves to reside profoundly in growing, understanding, relating, and caring.

Notes

1. LeCompte, M., & Dworkin, A. (1991). *Giving up on school: Student dropouts and teacher burnouts.* Thousand Oaks, CA: Corwin; U.S. Congress, Office of Technology Assessment. (1991). *Adolescent health, Vol. 1: Summary and policy options.* Washington, DC: U.S. Government Printing Office.

2. Marzano, R., & Marzano, J. (2003). The key to classroom management. *Educational Leadership, 61*(1), 6–13; Ferguson, R. (2002). *What doesn't meet the eye: Understanding and addressing racial disparities in high-achieving suburban schools.* Naperville, IL: North Central Regional Educational Laboratory.

3. I am not addressing, and my findings do not evidence, romantic relationships between teachers and students.

4. For more, see Farkas, S., & Johnson, J. (1997). *Kids these days: What Americans really think about the next generation.* New York: Public Agenda; Goleman, D. (1995). *Emotional intelligence.* New York: Bantam Books.

5. Phelan et al. assert: "It is not uncommon for low-achieving students to receive D's and F's in most classes while maintaining an A or B in an academic class that they describe as having a caring teacher" (pp. 698–699). Phelan, P., Davidson, A. L., & Cao, H. T. (1992). Speaking up: Students' perspectives on school. *Phi Delta Kappan, 73*(9), 695–704.

6. Erikson, E. H. (1968). *Identity: Youth and crisis.* New York: Norton.

7. Farkas & Johnson. (1997).

8. Csikszentmihalyi, M. (1987, Spring). The pressured world of adolescence. *Educational Horizons,* pp. 24–43.

9. Noam, G. G., Chandler, M., & LaLonde, C. (1995). Clinical-developmental psychology: Constructivism and social cognition in the study of psychological dysfunctions. In D. Cicchetti & D. Cohen (Eds.), *Handbook of developmental psychopathology* (Vol. 1, pp. 434–466). New York: Wiley (p. 442); Werner, E., & Smith, R. (1982). *Vulnerable but invincible: A longitudinal study of resilient children and youth.* New York: Adams, Bannister, and Cox.

10. Sizer, T. (1996). *Horace's hope: What works for the American high school.* Boston: Houghton Mifflin.

11. See, for example, the Coalition of Essential Schools' small schools project (http://www.essentialschools.org/pub/ces_docs/ssp/ssp.html) and San Diego City Schools, High School Reform Plan (http://www.sdcs.k12.ca.us/hsrenewal/index.html).

BETH BERNSTEIN-YAMASHIRO *is a grant director and former vice principal in the Long Beach Unified School District, Long Beach, California.*

Staff and youth can provide developmentally significant relationships for one another in out-of-school programs.

6

Emotional intelligence and staff training in after-school environments

Michelle Seligson, Marybeth MacPhee

THE GOAL OF applying relational psychology and emotional intelligence to professional development is to foster resonant relationships in which both participants grow. Such relationships offer the recognition, support, and acceptance necessary for developmental change.[1] Daloz has documented ways in which mentoring relationships between adults function as "holding environments" for the growth of both mentor and mentee.[2] We contend that adults can find a mix of support and challenge not only in interactions with colleagues and family, but also in relationships with children. In fact, caregiving poses a unique developmental challenge: to make meaningful connections with children that are marked by a sense of both responsibility and mutuality.

Dave is the director of a large after-school and summer program for school-age children living in a diverse metropolitan center.[3] He is a wizard at creating a safe haven for children who live in poverty and face violence in their neighborhoods, schools, and homes. Dave's ability to let each child in the program know that he cares about them magically transforms a less-than-ideal facility into a sanctuary. What makes Dave so unique in his patient, loving

NEW DIRECTIONS FOR YOUTH DEVELOPMENT, NO. 103, FALL 2004 © WILEY PERIODICALS, INC.

approach to the children in his program? Dave's father was very strict and pushed him hard to succeed. Dave and his siblings were not allowed to express much emotion in the family. Even so, Dave found the structure he experienced as he was growing up to be helpful when he started working with children because having clear boundaries gave the children a sense of safety. But he discovered something he did not know he had: his own nurturing ability, perhaps derived from his own longing for a more connected relationship with his dad.

Shioban took her job in another after-school program because of the immediate connection she made with her supervisor, the program's executive director. In the job interview, Mary, the supervisor, asked Shioban about herself and what she had done in her life that prepared her to work with children. Shioban felt immediately heard and knew that their working relationship in the program would be based on their similar values about what was important for the children. As this relationship grew through dealing with day-to-day issues, the two women developed a strong trust. Shioban never felt judged by Mary. They both learned from each other. Their relationship is critical to the reason she stays at the program, and Shioban is not sure that the values they share would be maintained by the larger organization if Mary were to leave.

Emotional intelligence

Many people think that Dave and Shioban's social and emotional skills are innate—you either have them or you do not—but Goleman argues that anyone can learn these skills with the right training and support.[4] The core concept of emotional intelligence is the ever-emerging process of self-awareness, where individuals are able to identify their emotions and manage them in various social environments. We view this capacity as an asset in child care because new insights in human development have highlighted the importance of children's social and emotional development and the process through which it helps them learn. As individuals grow and develop from infancy to adolescence and into adulthood, they enter and experience the world in terms of relationships.[5] Through relationships with parents and primary caregivers, infants, toddlers, and preschoolers learn the meaning of self and the value of self-regulation, an important part of social and emotional competence. A national committee on child mental health argues, "Children who do not achieve these age-appropriate social and emotional milestones face a far greater risk for early school failure."[6]

Expanding this perspective to older children, research and practice in psychology and education have argued that adult caregivers contribute to children's social and emotional needs, along with their physical needs, by engaging in quality interpersonal relationships. Identifying the characteristics of quality relationships for older children and youth, however, remains a challenge. Adults can enhance a child's self-esteem, foster social competence, and help build academic skills, but some researchers maintain that the ideal way to achieve these goals is elusive, idiosyncratic, and almost impossible to evaluate. Although empirical evidence clearly documents that children do better psychologically when they have at least one supportive relationship with an adult, Spencer contends that "we do not know *how* these relationships produce such significant effects."[7]

This chapter examines empirical and theoretical insights into how adults mobilize their inner resources and socioemotional aptitude to achieve good relationships with their coworkers and with the children and youth in their care and, more important, how other caregivers can learn these life skills. The integrative approach to professional development embedded in these questions forms the heart of the Bringing Yourself to Work project based at the Center for Research on Women at Wellesley College. The project focuses on training educators in self-awareness and relational practices to foster positive socioemotional learning environments for children. The theoretical foundation of this approach rests on increasing empirical and anecdotal evidence that success in life and in work is deeply connected with what Goleman calls "emotional literacy" with its five core aspects: self-awareness, the ability to handle emotions, self-motivation, empathic capacities, and social skills.[8]

In the work setting, Goleman contends that human contact is more essential than technology in accounting for success in business. He refers to the "low technology factors that make the difference between a successful training program and wasted organizational resources."[9] One of the most critical of these factors is the presence of people with emotional intelligence.

The following sections link empirical examples from pilot research and training sessions with after-school program directors in Massachusetts to highlight the relevance of self at work. Defining self is a complex task and beyond the scope of this chapter, but we situate our working definition within the scope of relational psychology, where one's sense of self, sense of agency, and place in the world develop from current and past relationships. We contextualize our discussion of self-awareness within the boundaries of the after-school work setting and offer a rationale for how educators can learn emotional intelligence.

Cohen applies this same concept to the success of children in school: "We all know that how we feel about ourselves and others can profoundly affect our ability to concentrate, to remember, to think, and to express ourselves. Many educators appreciate that we simply cannot separate 'academics' from the social and emotional lives of the classroom and the student. . . . Optimally, social and emotional learning (SEL) needs to be an integral part of children's education, in conjunction with linguistic, mathematical, aesthetic, kinesthetic, and ethical learning."[10]

Afterschool: Rational and relational views

The field of youth development has championed relational perspectives in its emphasis on the staff's capacity to connect with the youth. The presence of a supportive relationship with at least one adult makes a difference in the struggle to manage the social and emotional challenges at this stage. Practitioners in the child development field argue that it is important to establish these relationships before children reach adolescence. Young children thrive when sensitive, responsive caregivers provide generous amounts of attention as well as verbal and cognitive stimulation. Furthermore, the research shows that the combination of stability and skill creates the basis of quality in child care.[11]

Similarly, Spencer has found that skill and stability play a role in prevention programs. Adults who have "long-lasting and committed relationships" with youth in their communities bring care, trust, love, and acceptance into troubled environments.[12] More than the format or content of the intervention message, the leadership of a single adult made the program work successfully.[13] In research on adult youth workers in inner cities, McLaughlin and her colleagues observed that "it was less what the leaders did, and more the way they did it that seemed to have such a significant impact."[14] Successful youth leaders in the study emphasized the potential of the youth and the program to become resources for the community. More important, the leaders saw themselves as part of the community and learned from the youth in a joint effort to make a difference.

Some educators have innate leadership skills, while others can develop such skills with the kind of connection and support Shioban and Mary were able to develop in their program. As we show in the next section, successful after-school programs build into the program design opportunities for staff to reflect on what leads them to work with children and how those motivations affect their relationships with children.

In conducting visits to six after-school programs in Massachusetts during pilot research in 1998 and 1999, we found that programs emphasizing the personal development of adult educators have a more positive socioemotional climate than those that do not address adult development issues.[15] One of the participating after-school programs that work with adolescents provides a useful example of what we mean by positive socioemotional climate. This multicultural program, which serves forty adolescent girls, focuses on relationships. Because relationships are central to the program structure, adults create and take advantage of opportunities to talk with youth about personal matters individually or in small groups. The adults share their own lives, passions, and interests. When staff members break down the power dynamics that often exist between adults and youth, the teens can take a more active role in planning and implementing activities. This kind of participation offers opportunities for social and emotional learning and growth. Amy, an after-school student, noted, "They [the staff] don't have authority over us. It's not them and us—it's all *us*. They share what they are feeling and what's happening in their lives with us. It's nice to know that adults have feelings, too. Most adults never talk honestly about how their day went. They don't say how they feel about things."

Caren, one of the staff leaders, pointed out that the teens are sensitive about feeling judged and the program tries to provide a sanctuary from the kinds of pressures they face with grades at school or performance in sports or with peers. Staff have been able to facilitate this safe environment because they participate in adult sharing circles where they discuss memories of their own adolescence and issues that affect their capacity to help the girls. They are trained to know themselves and each other as individuals with strengths and weaknesses, fears and troubles, before they interact with the teens. This high level of relational awareness allows educators to better understand how differences in cultural background, communication styles, gender identity, and interest play out and how best to facilitate understanding across these differences.

The emphasis on authenticity and empathy helps group leaders create a sense of community and psychological safety for both the staff and the youth. Even when emotionally difficult issues arise—a fight at school, abuse at home, or an unexpected pregnancy, for example—staff leaders can be effective role models because they know how their own feelings and experience contribute to the energy of the group. When staff feel validated, supported, and connected, they can more readily help children feel validated, supported, and connected.

Creating connections across generations requires both self-awareness and other awareness, or empathy. Research on infant-caregiver interaction suggests that early relationships contribute to positive psychological development not only when complementary communication exchanges occur but also when the pair can successfully repair mismatches. Miller and Stiver take up this theme in their examination of healing connections in psychotherapy.[16] They see empathy and mutuality as essential components in maintaining emotional connections even when miscommunication occurs. Relational psychologists argue that individuals have an innate drive for human connection, but because problems linked to miscommunication have painful results, we protect ourselves by avoiding future connections. The freedom to express authentic emotions in balanced social relationships, conversely, allows individuals to thrive psychologically.

As the lens of developmental psychology widens to include relational capacity as a foundational part of human development, relationships are elevated as critical resources for growth and as the starting point for all educational endeavors. Projects such as the Reach Out to Schools Project (Wellesley College Stone Center), Educators for Social Responsibility, and Wellesley College Center for Research on Women's SEED (Seeking Educational Equity and Diversity) seminars aim to teach social competency through curriculum, but the embodied experience of connection serves as the most powerful tool for learning this approach. Knowledge of connection comes from gut feelings as much as verbal signals of understanding.

Emotions at work: Self-awareness with boundaries

Integrating relational practices at work calls for a reconceptualization of the structured roles of management and staff. Because the nature of these formerly hierarchical relationships in organizations has changed dramatically in recent years, an appeal for new paradigms of interpersonal relations at work has also grown.

To truly change the emotional climate of an organization, however, management must lead the way in setting new boundaries for the work role. Cooper and Sawaf argue that the key to successfully integrating the theory of emotional intelligence into everyday life is the issue of relevance.[17] Indulging in excessive self-exploration would transform work into therapy and coworkers into amateur therapists, yet suppressing self and feelings can contribute to volatile work environments. Advocates for emotional intelligence in schools find a balance in proposing that educators should have time and space at work for self-reflection. With the support of empathetic coworkers, educators are better able to recognize when emotion is controlling their actions, and they are able to learn how to channel that energy more creatively. When the adults are calm, they can teach children how to resolve their conflicts more responsibly and concentrate more effectively on their assignments.[18] Calm, however, does not mean being without emotion. The insights of relational psychology show that connections develop through empathy—feeling another person's pain or happiness and showing it.

When the interaction involves children, the issue extends beyond creating an effective work environment. From infancy through adolescence, these connections or relationships have direct impact on children's development and their success in school and in the rest of life. For that reason, there is an emerging body of literature advising educators and youth workers that these connections are a fundamental part of their work. Educators can share, according to their comfort level, feelings and stories to help children learn about the meaning and complexity of life in ways that objective academic lessons cannot.

The task of teaching and learning emotional, social, and relational skills to create quality human relationships in after-school programs is an emergent and complex process. Relationships between staff members and between staff and children enact ideas about power, cultural values, styles of communication, and personal experience that are often tricky to negotiate. For this reason, the discussion of what constitutes high-quality relationships requires exploration beyond the kind of behavioral suggestions listed in best-practice manuals. Leaders in this field integrate the kind of training required for state regulations with the kind of social and emotional training needed to create positive environments for staff and children. Research on relational psychology,[19] emotional intelligence, and socioemotional learning[20] has introduced new possibilities for enhancing quality relationships through self-awareness, self-control, and empathic listening.

In other work settings, leaders of the new flexible organizations have turned to innovative training programs to avoid or at least diminish the effects of postindustrial anxiety. At one level, experientially oriented programs expose coworkers to contrived situations of risk, such as ropes courses or Outward Bound–like experiences. The goal of these programs is to familiarize participants with feelings of vulnerability and fear to encourage a coping response that involves mutual trust and interdependence among coworkers with different roles in the organization. The social and emotional skills needed to survive the extreme physical risk of the training retreat serve as a model for succeeding in the workplace.[21]

Other organizations have turned to psychological experience training to achieve similar results. Emotional risk-taking programs use reflective surveys or group exercises to build the capacity for self-awareness, self-regulation, and emotional connections among participants. The Bringing Yourself to Work training workshops, for example, engage after-school program directors in experiential dyads and reflective exercises that focus on interpersonal relations at work. Researchers have measured the success of these interventions in terms of increased satisfaction at work, less anxiety, improved health of workers (including lower blood pressure), and increased efficiency and production of work, and they have found that the key to these successes is for individuals to learn how to manage their mental and emotional processes. These kinds of skills could have heightened value in after-school programs because interstaff relations model healthy communication and problem solving for children. The capacity to honestly listen to self and empathetically listen to others helps staff hear the essence of what children, coworkers, and parents need to improve the emotional climate of the program.[22]

Positive adult-youth relationships

The assertion that social-emotional learning is a vital part of human development hinges on the hypothesis that cognitive, emotional, and behavioral development are interconnected processes that begin in infancy and continue throughout life. In fostering the emotional development of adults, the Bringing Yourself to Work project complements other academic and professional training programs for after-school educators as well as school-based learning for children. At the root of theories in both relational psychology and socioemotional learning is a concern about how the weakening of community in modern American society affects individual development. Like the corner store and the neighborhood school, the rearing of children in a constant set of relationships bounded by home and community is rapidly fading from view. Amid all the changes children encounter as they grow and develop, the stability of these kinds of relational supports no longer can be taken for granted. Similarly, the workplace has replaced the neighborhood as a primary source of community, but restrictions on appropriate behavior at work have limited the degree to which individuals can express self and achieve mutuality in this setting.

Sociologist George Herbert Mead maintains that an individual's sense of self is acquired and sustained over time as it is "reflected in the judgment of others, both real and imagined."[23] In other words, our understanding of who we are requires the reflection gained from ongoing interaction with others in the community. Balanced psychological development suffers, however, when the dominant form of interaction in the society is extreme self-interest.

The recent emphasis on achievement in schools (for example, standardized testing) reflects a cultural value shift toward emphasizing competition and reward, at the expense of reciprocity and care. Adding elements of emotional intelligence and relational practices to staff training offers essential coping tools to the after-school practitioner to better define and value the role of caregiver.

Despite the personal and communal advantages of providing warmth, care, and support for the children, few programs explicitly identify healthy relationships as the core organizing principle in program design. Research on after-school programs often relies on what we refer to as proxies for relationship—references to particular aspects of quality that stand for adult-child relationships. Examples of such characteristic markers of good programs are relatively small adult-child ratios and group size, individual attention from caring adults, and low staff turnover.[24]

Program directors have a treasure chest of inner resources in their staff members, but it sometimes requires a little emotional digging to identify how these valuable feelings, experiences, and talents contribute to the group, including children. Creating specific times and activities for reflection and sharing among staff allows the participants to feel connection and disconnection in a structured way. In turn, this embodied experience establishes an internal barometer that can help staff in their relations with children and youth.

Notes

1. Brown, L. M., & Gilligan, C. (1992). *Meeting at the crossroads.* Cambridge, MA: Harvard University Press.
2. Daloz, L. A. (1986). *Effective teaching and mentoring.* San Francisco: Jossey Bass.
3. This name, like that of other study participants, is a pseudonym to maintain confidentiality in the research.
4. Goleman, D. (1995). *Emotional intelligence.* New York: Bantam Books.
5. Psychologists working at the Wellesley College Stone Center and the Harvard Project on Women's Psychology and Girls' Development have taken the lead in developing this perspective, which argues that mutuality rather than independence characterizes health development.
6. Child Mental Health Foundation. (2000). *A good beginning: Sending America's children to school with the social and emotional competence they need to succeed.* Bethesda, MD: National Institute of Mental Health.
7. Spencer, R. (2000). *Relationships that empower children for life: A report to the Stone Center directors.* Wellesley, MA: Wellesley College Stone Center.
8. Goleman, D. (1997). *Working with emotional intelligence.* New York: Bantam Books.
9. Goleman. (1997).
10. Cohen, J. (1999). *Educating hearts and minds: Social emotional learning and the passage into adolescence.* New York: Teachers College Press.
11. Belle, D. (1997). Varieties of self-care: A qualitative look at children's experiences in the after-school hours. *Merrill-Palmer Quarterly, 43*(2), 478–496.
12. Spencer. (2000).
13. In a study of eight after-school programs serving urban children in Chicago, Halpern (1992) found that staff who had been with a program longer knew the children better, knew more about their home environments, and were more likely to ask questions of the children if they started skipping the program. Unfortunately, staff longevity was atypical among the programs, with over 40 percent of the staff having been with the programs for less than a year.

This turnover was related to low staff salaries and the commonly held view that such work represented temporary employment rather than a career. Halpern, R. (1992). The role of after-school programs in the lives of inner-city children: A study of the Urban Youth Network. *Child Welfare League of America, 71*, 215–230.

14. Cited in Spencer. (2000).

15. One of the pressing issues in assessing quality in after-school programs is a high rate of staff turnover. Educators in this field lack the professional recognition, comprehensive training, and pay incentive of public school teachers but carry the burden of parents' and society's high expectations for program outcomes.

16. Miller, J. B., & Stiver, I. P. (1997). *The healing connection: How women form relationships in therapy and everyday life.* Boston: Beacon Press.

17. Cooper, R. K., & Sawaf, A. (1996). *Executive EQ: Emotional intelligence in leadership and organizations.* New York: Berkeley Publishing Group.

18. Cohen. (1999); Lantieri, L., & Patti, J. (1998). *Waging peace in our schools.* Boston: Beacon Press; Pianta, R. (1999). *Enhancing relationships between children and teachers.* Washington, DC: American Psychology Association.

19. Gilligan, C. (1996). The centrality of relationships in human development. In G. G. Noam & K. W. Fischer (Eds.), *Development and vulnerability in close relationships* (pp. 237–261). Mahwah, NJ: Erlbaum; Gilligan, C. (1989). Preface: Teaching Shakespeare's sister. In C. Gilligan, N. P. Lyons, & T. J. Hanmer (Eds.), *Making connections: The relational worlds of adolescent girls at Emma Willard School* (pp. 6–29). Cambridge, MA: Harvard University Press; Jordan, J. V. (1991). The meaning of mutuality. In J. V. Jordan, A. G. Kaplan, J. B. Miller, I. P. Stiver, & J. L. Surrey (Eds.), *Women's growth in connection* (pp. 81–96). New York: Guilford Press; Miller & Stiver. (1997).

20. Cohen. (1999).

21. Martin, E. (1994). *Flexible bodies: The role of immunity in American culture from the days of polio to the age of AIDS.* Boston: Beacon Press.

22. To be effective, a training model for after-school child care professionals needs to address the challenge of the elusive nature of emotion. Miller describes five "good things" that happen in relationships where psychological growth is happening for both people involved: (1) each person feels a greater sense of zest (vitality, energy); (2) each person feels more able to act and does act; (3) each person has a more accurate picture of herself or himself and the other person; (4) each person feels a greater sense of worth; and (5) each person feels more connected to the other person and feels a greater motivation for connections with other people beyond those in the specific relationship. Miller, J. B. (1986). *What do we mean by relationships?* Wellesley, MA: Wellesley College Centers for Research on Women.

23. Mead, G. H. (1967). *Mind, self, and society, from the standpoint of a social behaviorist.* Chicago: University of Chicago Press.

24. Alimbahai-Brown, Y. (1998, Aug. 21). Lack of respect leaves the young untouched. *Times Educational Supplement*, p. 10; Dresden, J., & Shetterley, K. R. (1997). Family child care and school-age programs: Today's friendly neighborhoods. *Dimensions of Early Childhood, 25*(1), 16–21; Halpern. (1992).

MICHELLE SELIGSON *is a researcher and author of several books on after-school program and policy, founder/director of the National Institute on Out-of-School Time at Wellesley College, and associate director/senior research scientists at the Wellesley Centers for Women.*

MARYBETH MACPHEE *is a cultural anthropologist and a postdoctoral fellow at Roger Williams University in Bristol, Rhode Island.*

Index

Academic achievement, 45–46
Adolescents: avoiding disconnection from, 25–26; bridging worlds of, 10; fear and coping of, 58–59; involvement in planning after-school activities, 76; myth of, 25; societal pressures on, 12–13
Adult-adult relationships, 10–11
Adult-youth relationships: benefits of, 1, 10, 19; challenges to, 32; childhood formation of, 74–75; core values of, 19; paradigm shift in, 1–2, 9; perception of, 9; students' need for, 64
After-school program staff: empathy of, 76–77; example of, 71–72; leadership of, 75; professional development of, 71–81, 82n.22; stability of, 75, 81–82n.13; turnover of, 82n.13–n.14
After-school programs: cross-referencing other domains with, 10–11; integrating emotional intelligence in, 77–79; and peer pressure, 76; reasons for student attendance in, 9; youth involvement in planning of, 76
Alcohol, 24
Anxiety, 58–60, 79
Attachment: benefits of, 11–12; importance of, 21–22; neurobiology and, 22–23; to primary caregiver, 10; and teacher-student relationship models, 48
Authenticity, 76
Authority, 63, 76
Autonomy, 12

Behavior: effect of parent-child relationship on, 23–24; parents' understanding of, 27

Belonging, 10
Bernstein-Yamashiro, B., 2, 7, 55
Blame, 27
Bowlby, J., 21, 22
Bringing Yourself to Work project, 73, 79, 80
Bullying, 19

Calmness, 78
Client-centered approach, 33
Cohen, J., 74
Collaborative relationship, 35
Communication recommendations, 27–28
Companionship, 39
Congruence, 34, 35
Cooper, R. K., 77

Daloz, L. A., 71
Depression, 19, 46
Developmental systems theory, 50
Dinners, 26
Diversity, 38–39
Dropout rates, 56
Drugs, 24

Educational policy, 56
Educators for Social Responsibility, 77
Emotional intelligence: core aspects of, 73; importance of, 74; integration of, 77–79; overview of, 72–73
Empathy, 33, 35, 76–77
Encouragement, 61
Environment, learning, 49, 51–52

Fear, 58–60
Feldman, S. S., 25–26
Fiore, N., 3, 5, 9
Fredriksen, K., 2, 6, 45

Notes for Contributors

New Directions for Youth Development: Theory, Practice, and Research is a quarterly publication focusing on current contemporary issues challenging the field of youth development. A defining focus of the journal is the relationship among theory, research, and practice. In particular, *NDYD* is dedicated to recognizing resilience as well as risk, and healthy development of our youth as well as the difficulties of adolescence. The journal is intended as a forum for provocative discussion that reaches across the worlds of academia, service, philanthropy, and policy.

In the tradition of the New Directions series, each volume of the journal addresses a single, timely topic, although special issues covering a variety of topics are occasionally commissioned. We welcome submissions of both volume topics and individual articles. All articles should specifically address the implications of theory for practice and research directions, and how these arenas can better inform one another. Articles may focus on any aspect of youth development; all theoretical and methodological orientations are welcome.

If you would like to be an *issue editor,* please submit an outline of no more than four pages (single spaced, 12 point type) that includes a brief description of your proposed topic and its significance along with a brief synopsis of individual articles (including tentative authors and a working title for each chapter).

If you would like to be an *author,* please submit first a draft of an abstract of no more than 1,500 words, including a two-sentence synopsis of the article; send this to the managing editor.

For all prospective issue editors or authors:

- Please make sure to keep accessibility in mind, by illustrating theoretical ideas with specific examples and explaining technical terms in nontechnical language. A busy practitioner who may not have an extensive research background should be well served by our work.

- Please keep in mind that references should be limited to twenty-five to thirty. Authors should make use of case examples to illustrate their ideas, rather than citing exhaustive research references. You may want to recommend two or three key articles, books, or Websites that are influential in the field, to be featured on a resource page. This can be used by readers who want to delve more deeply into a particular topic.
- All reference information should be listed as endnotes, rather than including author names in the body of the article or footnotes at the bottom of the page.

Please visit http://ndyd.org for more information.

Back Issue/Subscription Order Form

Copy or detach and send to:
Jossey-Bass, A Wiley Company, 989 Market Street, San Francisco, CA 94103-1741

Call or fax toll-free: Phone 888-378-2537 6:30AM – 3PM PST; Fax 888-481-2665

Back Issues: Please send me the following issues at $29 each
(Important: please include series initials and issue number, such as YD100.)

_____

_____

_____

$ _____   Total for single issues

$ _____

SHIPPING CHARGES: SURFACE	Domestic	Canadian
First Item	$5.00	$6.00
Each Add'l Item	$3.00	$1.50

For next-day and second-day delivery rates, call the number listed above.

Subscriptions: Please __start __renew my subscription to *New Directions for Youth Development* for the year 2_____ at the following rate:

U.S.	__Individual $80	__Institutional $170
Canada	__Individual $80	__Institutional $210
All Others	__Individual $104	__Institutional $244
U.S. Online Subscription		__Institutional $170
U.S. Print and Online Subscription		__Institutional $187

**For more information about online subscriptions visit
www.interscience.wiley.com**

$ _____   Total single issues and subscriptions (Add appropriate sales tax for your state for single issue orders. No sales tax for U.S. subscriptions. Canadian residents, add GST for subscriptions and single issues.)

__Payment enclosed (U.S. check or money order only)
__VISA __MC __AmEx #_____ Exp. Date _____

Signature _____ Day Phone _____
__ Bill Me (U.S. institutional orders only. Purchase order required.)

Purchase order # _____
     Federal Tax ID13559302   **GST 89102 8052**

Name _____

Address _____

_____

Phone _____ E-mail _____

Other Titles Available

NEW DIRECTIONS FOR YOUTH DEVELOPMENT: THEORY, PRACTICE, AND RESEARCH
Gil G. Noam, Editor-in-Chief

YD102 **Negotiation: Interpersonal Approaches to Intergroup Conflict**
Daniel L. Shapiro, Brooke E. Clayton
This issue considers the emotional complexities of intergroup conflict. The chapter authors examine the relational challenges that youth encounter in dealing with conflict and, combining innovative theory with ambitious practical application, identify conflict management strategies. These interventions have affected millions of youth across the continents.
ISBN 0-7879-7649-0

YD101 **After-School Worlds: Creating a New Social Space for Development and Learning**
Gil G. Noam
Showcases a variety of large-scale policy initiatives, effective institutional collaborations, and innovative programming options that produce high-quality environments in which young people are realizing their potential. Contributors underscore the conditions—from fostering interagency partnerships, to structuring organized out-of-school-time activities, to encouraging staff-student relationships—that lay the groundwork for positive youth development after school. At the same time, their examples illuminate the challenges for policymakers, researchers, and educators to redefine the field of afterschool as a whole, including the search for a shared lexicon, the push to preserve the character of afterschool as an intermediary space, and the need to create and further programs that are grounded in reliable research and that demonstrate success.
ISBN 0-7879-7304-1

YD100 **Understanding the Social Worlds of Immigrant Youth**
Carola Suárez-Orozco, Irina L. G. Todorova
This issue seeks to deepen understanding of the major social influences that shape immigrant youths' paths in their transition to the United States. The authors delve into a number of social worlds that can contribute to the positive development of immigrant youth. They also provide insight into sources of information about identity pathway options available to those youth. The chapters offer new data regarding the developmental opportunities that family roles and responsibilities, school contexts, community organizations, religious involvement and beliefs, gendered expectations, and media influences present.
ISBN 0-7879-7267-3

YD99   **Deconstructing the School-to-Prison Pipeline**
        Johanna Wald, Daniel J. Losen
        This issue describes how school policies can have the effect, if not
        the intent, of setting youths on the "prison track." It also identifies
        programs and policies that can help schools maintain safety and
        order while simultaneously reaching out to those students most in
        need of structure, education, and guidance. Offering a balanced per-
        spective, this issue begins to point the way toward less punitive, more
        effective, hopeful directions.
        ISBN 0-7879-7227-4

YD98   **Youth Facing Threat and Terror: Supporting Preparedness
        and Resilience**
        Robert D. Macy, Susanna Barry, Gil G. Noam
        Intended to help clinicians, youth and community workers, teachers,
        and parents to support resolution and recovery, this volume examines
        the effects of threat, stress, and traumatic events, including acts of ter-
        ror, on children and youth. It addresses not only the individual reper-
        cussions of threat but also a collective approach to threat. It also
        illustrates important ways to prevent traumatic situations from hav-
        ing lifelong, negative impacts. These methods involve providing
        immediate intervention and fostering safety as soon as a threatening
        incident has occurred as well as preparing children for future threats
        in ways that enhance feelings of safety rather than raise anxiety.
        ISBN 0-7879-7075-1

YD97   **When, Where, What, and How Youth Learn**
        Karen J. Pittman, Nicole Yohalem, Joel Tolman
        Acknowledging that young people learn throughout their waking
        hours, in a range of settings, and through a variety of means, this vol-
        ume presents practical advancements, theory development and new
        research in policies and infrastructures that support expanded defi-
        nitions of learning. Representing the perspectives of a broad range
        of scholars and practitioners, chapters explore ways to connect learn-
        ing experiences that happen inside and outside school buildings and
        during and after the school day. The contributors offer a compelling
        argument that communitywide commitments to learning are neces-
        sary if our nation's young people are to become problem free, fully
        prepared, and fully engaged.
        ISBN 0-7879-6848-X

YD96   **Youth Participation: Improving Institutions and Communities**
        Benjamin Kirshner, Jennifer L. O'Donoghue, Milbrey McLaughlin
        Explores the growing effort in youth organizations, community
        development, and schools and other public institutions to foster
        meaningful activities that empower adolescents to participate in deci-
        sion making that affects their lives and to take action on issues they
        care about. Pushing against long-held, culturally specific ideas about

adolescence as well as institutional barriers to youth involvement, the efforts of these organizations engaged in youth participation programs deserve careful analysis and support. This volume offers an assessment of the field, as well as specific chapters that chronicle efforts to achieve youth participation across a variety of settings and dimensions.
ISBN 0-7879-6339-9

YD95 **Pathways to Positive Development Among Diverse Youth**
Richard M. Lerner, Carl S. Taylor, Alexander von Eye
Positive youth development represents an emerging emphasis in developmental thinking that is focused on the incredible potential of adolescents to maintain healthy trajectories and develop resilience, even in the face of myriad negative influences. This volume discusses the theory, research, policy, and programs that take this strength-based, positive development approach to diverse youth. Examines theoretical ideas about the nature of positive youth development, and about the related concepts of thriving and well-being, as well as current and needed policy strategies, "best practice" in youth-serving programs, and promising community-based efforts to marshal the developmental assets of individuals and communities to enhance thriving among youth.
ISBN 0-7879-6338-0

YD94 **Youth Development and After-School Time: A Tale of Many Cities**
Gil G. Noam, Beth Miller
This issue looks at exciting citywide and cross-city initiatives in after-school time. It presents case studies of youth-related work that combines large-scale policy, developmental thinking, and innovative programming, as well as research and evaluation. Chapters discuss efforts of community-based organizations, museums, universities, schools, and clinics who are joining forces, sharing funding and other resources, and jointly creating a system of after-school care and education.
ISBN 0-7879-6337-2

YD93 **A Critical View of Youth Mentoring**
Jean E. Rhodes
Mentoring has become an almost essential aspect of youth development and is expanding beyond the traditional one-to-one, volunteer, community-based mentoring. This volume provides evidence of the benefits of enduring high-quality mentoring programs, as well as apprenticeships, advisories, and other relationship-based programs that show considerable promise. Authors examine mentoring in the workplace, teacher-student interaction, and the mentoring potential of student advising programs. They also take a critical look at the importance of youth-adult relationships and how a deeper

understanding of these relationships can benefit youth mentoring. This issue raises important questions about relationship-based interventions and generates new perspectives on the role of adults in the lives of youth.
ISBN 0-7879-6294-5

YD92 **Zero Tolerance: Can Suspension and Expulsion Keep Schools Safe?**
Russell J. Skiba, Gil G. Noam
Addressing the problem of school violence and disruption requires thoughtful understanding of the complexity of the personal and systemic factors that increase the probability of violence, and designing interventions based on that understanding. This inaugural issue explores the effectiveness of zero tolerance as a tool for promoting school safety and improving student behavior and offers alternative strategies that work.
ISBN 0-7879-1441-X

NEW DIRECTIONS FOR YOUTH DEVELOPMENT IS NOW AVAILABLE ONLINE AT WILEY INTERSCIENCE

What is Wiley InterScience?

Wiley InterScience is the dynamic online content service from John Wiley & Sons delivering the full text of over 300 leading scientific, technical, medical, and professional journals, plus major reference works, the acclaimed *Current Protocols* laboratory manuals, and even the full text of select Wiley print books online.

What are some special features of Wiley InterScience?

Wiley InterScience Alerts is a service that delivers table of contents via e-mail for any journal available on Wiley InterScience as soon as a new issue is published online.
Early View is Wiley's exclusive service presenting individual articles online as soon as they are ready, even before the release of the compiled print issue. These articles are complete, peer-reviewed, and citable.
CrossRef is the innovative multi-publisher reference linking system enabling readers to move seamlessly from a reference in a journal article to the cited publication, typically located on a different server and published by a different publisher.

How can I access Wiley InterScience?

Visit http://www.interscience.wiley.com

Guest Users can browse Wiley InterScience for unrestricted access to journal Tables of Contents and Article Abstracts, or use the powerful search engine.
Registered Users are provided with a *Personal Home Page* to store and manage customized alerts, searches, and links to favorite journals and articles. Additionally, Registered Users can view free Online Sample Issues and preview selected material from major reference works.
Licensed Customers are entitled to access full-text journal articles in PDF, with select journals also offering full-text HTML.

How do I become an Authorized User?

Authorized Users are individuals authorized by a paying Customer to have access to the journals in Wiley InterScience. For example, a university that subscribes to Wiley journals is considered to be the Customer. Faculty, staff and students authorized by the university to have access to those journals in Wiley InterScience are Authorized Users. Users should contact their Library for information on which Wiley journals they have access to in Wiley InterScience.

ASK YOUR INSTITUTION ABOUT WILEY INTERSCIENCE TODAY!